EMERGING INFECTIOUS DISEASES FROM THE GLOBAL TO THE LOCAL PERSPECTIVE

A Summary
of a Workshop of the
Forum on Emerging Infections

Jonathan R. Davis and Joshua Lederberg, *Editors*

Board on Global Health

INSTITUTE OF MEDICINE

NATIONAL ACADEMY PRESS
Washington, D.C.

NATIONAL ACADEMY PRESS • 2101 Constitution Avenue, N.W. • Washington, DC 20418

NOTICE: The project that is the subject of this workshop summary was approved by the Governing Board of the National Research Council, whose members are drawn from the councils of the National Academy of Sciences, the National Academy of Engineering, and the Institute of Medicine.

Support for this project was provided by the U.S. Department of Health and Human Services' National Institutes of Health, Centers for Disease Control and Prevention, and U.S. Food and Drug Administration; U.S. Department of Defense; U.S. Department of State; U.S. Department of Veterans Affairs; Abbott Laboratories; American Society for Microbiology; Bristol-Myers Squibb Company; Burroughs Wellcome Fund; Eli Lilly & Company; Glaxo Wellcome; F. Hoffmann-La Roche, AG; Pfizer, Inc.; SmithKline Beecham Corporation; and Wyeth-Ayerst Laboratories. The views presented are those of the editors and workshop participants and are not necessarily those of the funding organizations.

This report is based on the proceedings of a workshop that was sponsored by the Forum on Emerging Infections. It is prepared in the form of a workshop summary by and in the name of the editors, with the assistance of staff and consultants, as an individually authored document. Sections of the workshop summary not specifically attributed to an individual reflect the views of the editors and not those of the Forum on Emerging Infections. The content of those sections is based on the presentations and the discussions that took place during the workshop.

International Standard Book Number 0-309-07184-4

Additional copies of this report are available for sale from the National Academy Press, 2101 Constitution Avenue, N.W., Box 285, Washington, DC 20055. Call (800) 624-6242 or (202) 334-3313 (in the Washington metropolitan area), or visit the NAP's on-line bookstore at **www.nap.edu.** The full text is available on line at **www.nap.edu.**

For information about the Institute of Medicine, visit the IOM home page at **www. iom.edu.**

COVER: The background for the cover of this workshop summary is a photograph of a batik designed and printed specifically for the Malaysian Society of Parasitology and Tropical Medicine. The print contains drawings of various parasites and insects; it is used with the kind permission of the Society.

*"Knowing is not enough; we must apply.
Willing is not enough; we must do."*

—Goethe

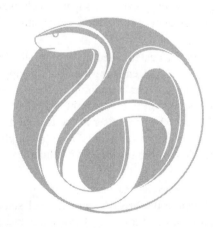

INSTITUTE OF MEDICINE

Shaping the Future for Health

THE NATIONAL ACADEMIES

National Academy of Sciences
National Academy of Engineering
Institute of Medicine
National Research Council

The **National Academy of Sciences** is a private, nonprofit, self-perpetuating society of distinguished scholars engaged in scientific and engineering research, dedicated to the furtherance of science and technology and to their use for the general welfare. Upon the authority of the charter granted to it by the Congress in 1863, the Academy has a mandate that requires it to advise the federal government on scientific and technical matters. Dr. Bruce M. Alberts is president of the National Academy of Sciences.

The **National Academy of Engineering** was established in 1964, under the charter of the National Academy of Sciences, as a parallel organization of outstanding engineers. It is autonomous in its administration and in the selection of its members, sharing with the National Academy of Sciences the responsibility for advising the federal government. The National Academy of Engineering also sponsors engineering programs aimed at meeting national needs, encourages education and research, and recognizes the superior achievements of engineers. Dr. William A. Wulf is president of the National Academy of Engineering.

The **Institute of Medicine** was established in 1970 by the National Academy of Sciences to secure the services of eminent members of appropriate professions in the examination of policy matters pertaining to the health of the public. The Institute acts under the responsibility given to the National Academy of Sciences by its congressional charter to be an adviser to the federal government and, upon its own initiative, to identify issues of medical care, research, and education. Dr. Kenneth I. Shine is president of the Institute of Medicine.

The **National Research Council** was organized by the National Academy of Sciences in 1916 to associate the broad community of science and technology with the Academy's purposes of furthering knowledge and advising the federal government. Functioning in accordance with general policies determined by the Academy, the Council has become the principal operating agency of both the National Academy of Sciences and the National Academy of Engineering in providing services to the government, the public, and the scientific and engineering communities. The Council is administered jointly by both Academies and the Institute of Medicine. Dr. Bruce M. Alberts and Dr. William A. Wulf are chairman and vice chairman, respectively, of the National Research Council

FORUM ON EMERGING INFECTIONS

JOSHUA LEDERBERG (*Chair*), Sackler Foundation Scholar, The Rockefeller University, New York, New York

VINCENT I. AHONKHAI, Vice President and Director, Anti-Infectives and Biologicals, SmithKline Beecham Corporation, Collegeville, Pennsylvania

STEVEN J. BRICKNER, Manager of Medicinal Chemistry, Central Research Division, Pfizer, Inc., Groton, Connecticut

GAIL H. CASSELL, Vice President for Infectious Diseases Research, Drug Discovery Research, and Clinical Investigation, Eli Lilly & Company, Indianapolis, Indiana

GARY CHRISTOPHERSON, Principal Deputy Assistant Secretary for Health Affairs and Senior Advisor for Force Health Protection, U.S. Department of Defense Reserve Affairs, Washington, D.C.

GORDON H. DeFRIESE, Director and Professor of Social Medicine, Epidemiology, Health Policy, and Administration, Sheps Center for Health Services Research, University of North Carolina, Chapel Hill, North Carolina

CEDRIC E. DUMONT, Medical Director, Office of Medical Services, U.S. Department of State, Washington, D.C.

JESSE GOODMAN, Acting Deputy Director, Center for Biologics Evaluation and Research, U.S. Food and Drug Administration, Washington, D.C.

RENU GUPTA, Head of U.S. Research and Development, and Head of Global Cardiovascular, Metabolic, and Endocrine G.I Disorders, Novartis Pharmaceuticals, East Hanover, New Jersey

MARGARET A. HAMBURG, Assistant Secretary for Planning and Evaluation, U.S. Department of Health and Human Services, Washington, D.C.

CAROLE A. HEILMAN, Director, Division of Microbiology and Infectious Disease, National Institute of Allergy and Infectious Diseases, National Institutes of Health, Bethesda, Maryland

JAMES M. HUGHES, Assistant Surgeon General, and Director, National Center for Infectious Diseases, Centers for Disease Control and Prevention, Atlanta, Georgia

SAMUEL L. KATZ, Wilburt C. Davison Professor, Department of Pediatrics, Duke University Medical Center; Undersecretary for Health, Veterans Health Administration, U.S. Department of Veterans Affairs, Washington, D.C.

MARCELLE LAYTON, Bureau of Communicable Diseases, New York City Department of Health, New York, New York

CARLOS LOPEZ, Research Fellow, Research Acquisitions, Eli Lilly Research Laboratories, Indianapolis, Indiana

STEPHEN S. MORSE, Professor of Epidemiology, Columbia University School of Public Health, New York, New York

MICHAEL T. OSTERHOLM, Chairman and Chief Executive Officer, Infectious Control Advisory Network, Eden Prairie, Minnesota

MARC RUBIN, Vice President of Infectious Diseases Therapeutic Development Group, Glaxo Wellcome, Research Triangle Park, North Carolina

DAVID M. SHLAES, Vice President, Infectious Disease Research, Wyeth-Ayerst Research, Pearl River, New York .

JANET SHOEMAKER, Director, Public Affairs, American Society for Microbiology, Washington, D.C.

JOHN D. SIEGFRIED, Deputy Vice-President, Science and Regulatory Affairs, Pharmaceutical Research and Manufacturers of America, Washington, D.C.

P. FREDERICK SPARLING, Chair of Medicine, University of North Carolina at Chapel Hill, and President, Infectious Diseases Society of America, Washington, D.C.

C. DOUGLAS WEBB, JR., Senior Medical Director, Infectious Diseases Global Marketing, Bristol-Myers Squibb, Princeton, New Jersey

CATHERINE E. WOTEKI, Undersecretary for Food and Safety, U.S. Department of Agriculture, Washington, D.C.

Liaisons to the Forum

ENRIQUETA C. BOND, President, Burroughs Wellcome Fund, Morrisville, North Carolina

NANCY CARTER-FOSTER, Director, Program for Emerging Infections and HIV/AIDS, U.S. Department of State, Washington, D.C.

PATRICK W. KELLEY, Colonel, U.S. Army, and Director, Division of Preventive Medicine, Walter Reed Army Institute of Research, Washington, D.C.

EDWARD MCSWEEGAN, Division of Microbiology and Infectious Diseases, National Institute of Allergy and Infectious Diseases, National Institutes of Health, Bethesda, Maryland

STEPHEN M. OSTROFF, Acting Deputy Director, and Associate Director for Epidemiologic Science, National Center for Infectious Diseases, Centers for Disease Control and Prevention, Atlanta, Georgia

GARY ROSELLE, Program Director for Infectious Disease, Veterans Health Administration, U.S. Department of Veterans Affairs, Cincinnati, Ohio

JAMES M. SIGG, Contract Liaison Officer, Office of Management and Contracts, Centers for Biologics Evaluation and Research, U.S. Food and Drug Administration, Washington, D.C.

FRED TENOVER, Chief, Nosocomial Pathogens Laboratory Branch, National Center for Infectious Diseases, Centers for Disease Control and Prevention, Atlanta, Georgia

KAYE WACHSMUTH, Deputy Administrator, Office of Public Health and Science, Food Safety Inspection Service, U.S. Department of Agriculture, Washington, D.C.

Study Staff

JONATHAN R. DAVIS, Senior Program Officer
VIVIAN P. NOLAN, Research Associate

NICOLE AMADO, Project Assistant
THELMA COX, Project Assistant
KATHI HANNA, *Consultant*
MICHAEL HAYES, *Copy Editor*

Division Staff

JUDITH R. BALE, Director, Board on Global Health
ANDREW M. POPE, Director, Board on Health Sciences Policy
SARAH PITLUCK, Research Assistant
ALDEN CHANG, Project Assistant
ANDREA L. COHEN, Financial Associate
CARLOS GABRIEL, Financial Associate

REVIEWERS

All presenters at the workshop have reviewed and approved their respective sections of this report for accuracy. In addition, this workshop summary has been reviewed in draft form by independent reviewers chosen for their diverse perspectives and technical expertise, in accordance with procedures approved by the National Research Council's Report Review Committee. The purpose of this independent review is to provide candid and critical comments that will assist the Institute of Medicine (IOM) in making the published workshop summary as sound as possible and to ensure that the workshop summary meets institutional standards. The review comments and draft manuscript remain confidential to protect the integrity of the deliberative process.

The Forum and IOM thank the following individuals for their participation in the review process:

Kenneth Bart, M.D., M.P.H., Director, Graduate School of Public Health, College of Health and Human Services, San Diego Sate University, San Diego, California

Joel Breman, M.D., D.T.P.H., Deputy Director, Division of International Training and Research, Fogarty International Center, National Institutes of Health, Bethesda, Maryland

Walter R. Dowdle, Ph.D., Task Force for Child Survival and Development, Decatur, Georgia

Nancy B. Mock, Dr.P.H., Director and Associate Professor of International Health, Tulane University, New Orleans, Louisiana

Patricia Quinlisk, M.D., Medical Director, Iowa Department of Health, Des Moines, Iowa

Robert E. Shope, M.D., Professor, Department of Pathology, University of Texas Medical Branch, Galveston, Texas

Although the reviewers listed above have provided many constructive comments and suggestions, they were not asked to endorse the conclusions or recommendations nor did they see the final draft of the report before its release. The review of this report was overseen by Adel A. F. Mahmoud, M.D., Ph.D., President, Merck Vaccines, Merck and Co., Inc., Whitehouse Station, New Jersey, who was responsible for making certain that an independent examination of this report was carried out in accordance with institutional procedures and that all review comments were carefully considered. Responsibility for the final content of this report rests entirely with the editors.

Preface

The Forum on Emerging Infections was created in 1996 in response to a request from the Centers for Disease Control and Prevention and the National Institutes of Health. The goal of the Forum is to provide structured opportunities for representatives from academia, industry, professional and interest groups, and government[*] to examine and discuss scientific and policy issues that are of shared interest and that are specifically related to research and prevention, detection, and management of emerging infectious diseases. In accomplishing this task, the Forum provides the opportunity to foster the exchange of information and ideas, identify areas in need of greater attention, clarify policy issues by enhancing knowledge and identifying points of agreement, and inform decision makers about science and policy issues. The Forum seeks to illuminate issues rather than resolve them directly; hence, it does not provide advice or recommendations on any specific policy initiative pending before any agency or organization. Its strengths are the diversity of its membership and the commitment of individual members expressed throughout the activities of the Forum.

A critical part of the work of the Forum is a series of workshops. The first of these, held in February 1997, addressed the theme of public- and private-sector collaboration (IOM, 1997). The second workshop took place in July 1997 and explored aspects of antimicrobial resistance (IOM, 1998). The third workshop (IOM, 2000a) examined the implications of managed care systems and the

---

[*]Representatives of federal agencies serve in an *ex officio* capacity. An *ex officio* member of a group is one who is a member automatically by virtue of holding a particular office or membership in another body.

ix

ability to address emerging infectious diseases in the age of managed care. The fourth workshop (IOM, 2000b) examined the core capacities of the public and private health sectors in emerging infectious disease surveillance and response. The fifth workshop, held in October 1999, which this document summarizes, examined the international aspects of emerging infections and the forces that drive these diseases to prominence from the global to the local levels. The topic of zoonotic diseases was the focus of the Forum's sixth workshop, which was held in June 2000. The summary of that workshop is in production. The next workshop sponsored by the Forum will address factors surrounding viral disease eradication.

ABOUT THE WORKSHOP

In recent years, emerging infections have captured increased attention internationally. This comes at a time when other diseases are gaining in importance. In an effort to increase our knowledge and understanding of the current and probable future public health significance of emerging infections internationally, the Institute of Medicine's Forum on Emerging Infections hosted a 2-day workshop on October 28 and 29, 1999, titled "International Aspects of Emerging Infections." The goal of the workshop was to collect new information on this topic from public health practitioners, academicians, and policy makers at the global, regional, national, and local levels from various geographical areas. Their presentations focused on the interplay among emerging infections, economics and trade, public health policies, population and demography, strategic planning and resource allocation, and infrastructure and capacity at their positions of practice. Panel discussions then focused on the interaction of these factors with infectious disease surveillance and response, communication and coordination, and research and training needs with recognition of the lessons and mistakes learned in the process and identification of novel approaches and obstacles at each level. Through the presentations and discussions, we hope to gain new insight into

• the forces that drive the policies of governments and international organizations;
• the ways in which diseases are prioritized; and
• the strengths and weaknesses of past and current local, national, and multinational efforts to effectively bring nations and international organizations closer together to mitigate the impacts of emerging infections.

Early-on during the workshop, it was clear that the infrastructure and level of support for surveillance, research, and training on emerging infectious diseases varied widely across geographic regions. For example, in many countries a shrinking number of trained infectious disease specialists was cited. The latter point was accentuated while developing the workshop as some of the foreign scientists invited to make presentations were unavailable owing to exigent schedules and demanding workloads for the qualified few, in addition to difficulty in obtaining government permission to travel and technological obstacles to effective communication. Consequently, although the presentations were rich and wide-ranging, the workshop did not support a comprehensive and balanced treatment of issues across regions.

ORGANIZATION OF WORKSHOP SUMMARY

This report of the Forum-sponsored workshop is prepared in the form of a workshop summary by and in the name of the editors, with the assistance of staff and consultants, as an individually authored document. Sections of the workshop summary not specifically attributed to an individual reflect the views of the editors and not those of the Forum on Emerging Infections or its sponsors. The contents of the unattributed sections are based on the presentations and discussions that took place during the workshop.

The workshop summary is organized as a topic-by-topic description of the presentations and discussions. Its purpose is to present lessons from relevant experience, delineate a range of pivotal issues and their respective problems, and put forth some potential responses as described by the workshop participants. The Summary and Assessment chapter discusses the core messages that emerged from the speakers' presentations and the ensuing discussions. Chapter 1 is an introduction and overview of the international perspective on confronting emerging infections. Chapters 2 to 5 begin with overviews provided by the editors, followed by the edited presentations made by the invited participants. Appendix A is a glossary and list of acronyms useful to the reader. Appendix B presents the workshop agenda. A list of workshop participants is found in Appendix C. Forum members and staff biographies are presented in Appendix D.

Although this workshop summary provides an account of the individual presentations, it also reflects an important aspect of the Forum philosophy. The workshop functions as a dialogue among representatives from different sectors and presents their beliefs on which areas may merit further attention. However, the reader should be aware that the material presented here expresses the views and opinions of those participating in the workshop and not the deliberations of a formally constituted Institute of Medicine study committee. These proceedings summarize only what participants stated in the workshop and are not intended to be an exhaustive exploration of the subject matter.

ACKNOWLEDGMENTS

The Forum on Emerging Infections and the Institute of Medicine (IOM) wish to express their warmest appreciation to the individuals and organizations who gave valuable time to provide information and advice to the Forum through participation in the workshop.

The Forum is indebted to the IOM staff who contributed during the course of the workshop and the production of this workshop summary. On behalf of the Forum, I gratefully acknowledge the efforts led by Jonathan Davis, study director for the Forum and coeditor of this report, who dedicated much effort and time to developing this workshop's agenda and for his thoughtful and insightful approach and skill in translating the workshop proceedings and discussion into this workshop summary. I would also like to thank the following IOM staff for their valuable contributions to this activity: Vivian Nolan assisted with the development of the workshop agenda, Thelma Cox assisted with editing various sections of the workshop summary list and provided comprehensive administrative support and Nicole Amado assisted in developing the glossary and acronyms in Appendix A. Other IOM staff also provided invaluable help: Sue Barron, Clyde Behney, Claudia Carl, Michael Edington, Carlos Gabriel, and Andrew Pope. Kathi Hanna, a consultant and technical writer contributed significantly to writing many sections of the workshop summary. The extensive commentary and suggestions made by the copy editor, Michael Hayes, are gratefully acknowledged.

Finally, the Forum also thanks sponsors that supported this activity. Financial support for this project was provided by the U.S. Department of Health and Human Services' National Institutes of Health, Centers for Disease Control and Prevention, and the U.S. Food and Drug Administration; U.S. Department of Defense; U.S. Department of State; U.S. Department of Veterans Affairs; Abbott Laboratories; American Society for Microbiology; Bristol-Myers Squibb Company; Burroughs Wellcome Fund; Eli Lilly & Company; Glaxo Wellcome; F. Hoffmann-La Roche AG; Pfizer; SmithKline Beecham Corporation; and Wyeth-Ayerst Laboratories. The views presented in this workshop summary are those of the editors and workshop participants and are not necessarily those of the funding organizations.

Joshua Lederberg
Chair

Contents

EMERGING INFECTIOUS DISEASES FROM THE GLOBAL TO THE LOCAL PERSPECTIVE

Summary and Assessment

Joshua Lederberg, Ph.D.
Nobel Laureate and Sackler Foundation Scholar,
The Rockefeller University

In October 1999, the Forum on Emerging Infections of the Institute of Medicine convened a 2-day workshop titled "International Aspects of Emerging Infections." Key representatives from the international community explored the forces that drive emerging infectious diseases to prominence. Representatives from the Americas, Africa, Asia and the Pacific, and Europe made formal presentations and engaged in panel discussions. Summaries of the formal presentations can be found in Chapters 1 through 5 of this report. The topics addressed during this conference cover a wide range of issues, including trends in the incidence of infectious diseases around the world, descriptions of the wide variety of factors that contribute to the emergence and reemergence of these diseases, efforts to coordinate surveillance activities and responses within and across borders, and the resource, research, and international needs that remain to be addressed. This section of the report summarizes the issues raised during the 2-day meeting and suggests an agenda for future action.

EMERGING INFECTIONS: THE GLOBAL PICTURE

In his keynote address, David Heymann, Executive Director of Communicable Diseases for the World Health Organization (WHO), described the global proportions of infectious diseases. Infectious diseases are undergoing a global resurgence and threaten the health of everyone. They remain the world's greatest killer of children and young adults, accounting for more than 13 million deaths a

1

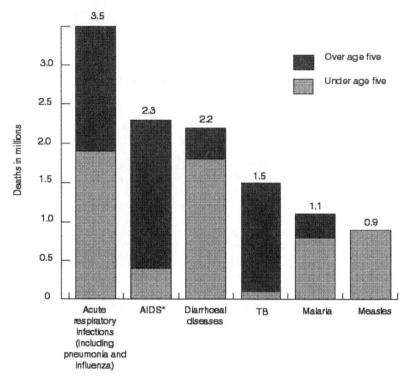

FIGURE 1 Leading infectious killers; millions of deaths worldwide, all ages, 1998. *HIV-positive people who died with TB have been included among AIDS deaths. SOURCE: WHO, 1999.

year and half of all deaths in developing countries, with six diseases causing 90 percent of deaths from infectious diseases: pneumonia, tuberculosis (TB), diarrheal diseases, malaria, measles, and human immunodeficiency virus infection (HIV)/AIDS (Figure 1).

Even though most deaths from infectious diseases occur in developing countries, no region of the world is free from concern. In 1996 and 1997 alone, every continent experienced a large outbreak of some type of infectious disease, from Lyme disease in North America to Ross River virus in Australia (Figure 2). Therefore, it is in the best interest of all countries to support global initiatives to control infectious diseases.

In addition, the growing rise and spread of antimicrobial resistance is of increasing concern in developed countries as the inappropriate use of antibiotics goes unchecked. Moreover, increasing numbers of international travelers provide a vehicle for the rapid spread of microbes resistant to antimicrobial agents. For example, in 1995 two different clones of multidrug-resistant *Streptococcus pneumoniae* were first identified in Spain, and within 2 months the strains had been found in Croatia, France, Mexico, Portugal, Korea, South Africa, and the United States (Figure 3).

The reemergence of infectious diseases once thought to be under control or eliminated is also a growing concern. For example, dengue fever is a disease of humans in tropical and subtropical regions caused by the dengue virus, which is transmitted from human to human by the bite of an infected *Aedes* mosquito. In the past decade, countries in the Americas, Southeast Asia, and Western Pacific have witnessed a resurgence of dengue fever and its most serious manifestation, dengue hemorrhagic fever (Figure 4). Yet, the rise of dengue is not the only concern of the global population public health community. In 1996, outbreaks of polio in Albania, Greece, and Yugoslavia, and more recently in Haiti and the Dominican Republic, demonstrated that when immunization practices and disease surveillance are neglected, diseases can easily be reintroduced into countries once free of a malady.

Financial Costs of Infectious Diseases

Beyond the human suffering, the financial costs of infectious diseases are great, especially for developing countries (Table 1). The economic burden of malaria alone has cost Africa billions of dollars over the past decade. When infectious diseases are not controlled, they take a tremendous toll on the econo port of goods. Although they are not always high on the list of causes of mortality, infectious diseases may be high on the list of causes of economic morbidity:

• In 1994, the panic over plague in India cost the country an estimated $1.8 billion in lost tourist income and trade.

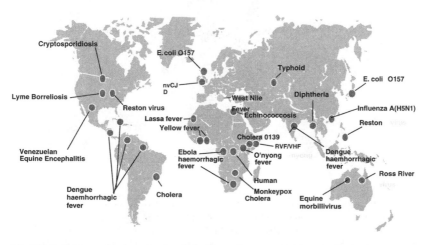

FIGURE 2 Emerging/reemerging infectious diseases, 1996 and 1997. SOURCE: WHO/CDS, 1999.

TABLE 1 Infectious Diseases and Their Costs to Economies

Year(s)	Country	Disease	Cost (millions of US$)
1990 to 1998	United Kingdom	Bovine Spongiform Encephalopathy	>5,740
1991	Peru	Cholera	770
1991	India	Plague	1,800
1994	India	Tuberculosis	>1,000
1997	Tanzania	Cholera	36
1997 to 1998	Thailand	HIV/AIDS	2,500

SOURCE: Workshop presentation by David Heymann, World Health Organization, 1999.

• In 1996 the European Union banned the worldwide export of British beef in response to fears about bovine spongiform encephalopathy (so-called mad cow disease).

• In 1998 the European Union erected trade barriers because of a cholera outbreak in East Africa, where the disease is endemic.

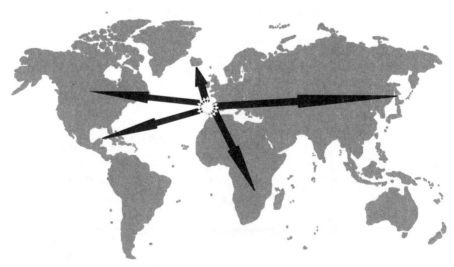

FIGURE 3 *Streptococcus pneumoniae:* probable spread of two multi-resistant clones in a two-month period. First clone in Spain, subsequently in Croatia, France, Mexico, Portugal, Republic of Korea, South Africa, and the United States. Different clone, first seen in Spain, and subsequently in Iceland. SOURCE: WHO Report WHO/CDS/BVI/95.7.

Americas Region

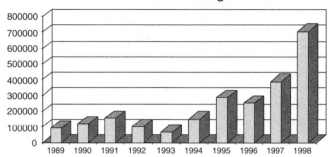

South-East Asia Region

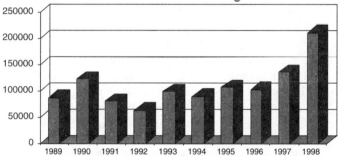

Western Pacific Region

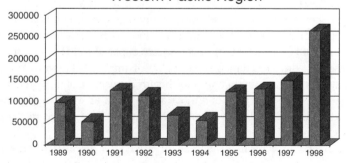

FIGURE 4 Resurgence of dengue fever and dengue hemorrhagic fever; number of cases. SOURCE: WHO/CDS, 1999.

Additionally, the economic and societal costs of controlling infectious diseases are directly proportional to the response time to control the disease. For example, the emergence of HIV/AIDS has prompted a global resurgence of tuberculosis (TB), especially multidrug-resistant TB (MDR-TB). Treatment costs for TB can vary between $15 and $40 per person to achieve a complete cure, whereas treatment costs for MDR-TB are $3,000 per person. Considering that total spending for health care in some of the poorest countries in the world is less than $7 per person per year, the increased costs associated with a delayed response to disease control are beyond the reach of the poorest countries. Not only does treatment become impossible as economic and societal costs increase, but infectious disease control is often neglected, as are disease prevention efforts.

Infectious Diseases and Human Rights

In some countries the issues of the spread and control of infectious diseases are interwoven with concerns about human rights. In some Asian countries large populations migrate to neighboring countries. However, if an immigrant contracts HIV or even viral hepatitis, the person is frequently sent back to the country of origin, a place from which he or she might have fled. Thus, some are hesitant to seek medical care and often go "underground," spreading the disease even further. The Hong Kong Special Administration Region counters this possibility by ensuring that individuals who are positive for HIV are offered a full range of services, with the assurance that they will not be deported or detained if they seek medical care.

Infectious diseases among incarcerated individuals are also on the rise worldwide. In Russia, 42 percent of all TB cases are detected in the prison population. Every year the system incarcerates 300,000 otherwise healthy Russians and releases another 300,000, most of whom will have been exposed to TB during their incarcerations. Among these individuals, approximately 10 percent develop active disease and 80 percent carry the TB bacterium in a latent state. Approximately 40 percent of those patients are exposed to MDR strains. Among the amplifiers of drug resistance is the delay of implementation of directly observed treatment (short course) and poor health care services in Russian prisons. Tragically, the MDR-TB crisis is almost at the point at which the disease may never be controlled there unless second line drugs are introduced into the prison system (see Chapter 5).

Thus, efforts to control the spread of infectious diseases often encounter national and regional issues to which the international community is sometimes hesitant or unable to respond. Better surveillance for diseases in refugee and prison populations is needed to detect infectious agents, institute therapy or control strategies, and prevent or mitigate the impact and further spread of contagion.

FACTORS IN EMERGENCE OF
INFECTIOUS DISEASES

Specific factors are responsible for the emergence of infectious diseases. With proper epidemiological investigations and laboratory surveillance, the determinants of disease outbreaks can be identified, as most emerging infections (even those resistant to antimicrobial agents) usually originate in one location and then disseminate to new areas. Complacency about vaccination and antibiotic use, however, and the lack of investment in surveillance and control programs have exacerbated the spread of many diseases. Climate variability and natural disasters also play a role in the emergence of many infectious diseases. For example, the traditional meningitis A belt was limited to Saharan Africa. Recently, however, there have been epidemics occurring farther south, in Uganda, Kenya, and Tanzania, and these are likely related to droughts in those areas. In some countries, devastating earthquakes and floods have contributed to outbreaks of cholera, malaria, TB, and diarrheal diseases.

In the past 20 years a number of global activities have resulted in an increase in the level of spread of infectious microbes and have promoted the emergence of diseases and epidemics (Table 2). Many of these factors lie outside the purview of the health sector, making it difficult to mitigate their impact on the transmission of infectious diseases and requiring coordinated approaches among various sectors of society for successful control. For example, economic and environmental policies can have direct and negative effects on the emergence and spread of infectious diseases. Deforestation and changes in land and water use can also affect disease patterns, triggering outbreaks of parasitic or other infectious diseases.

TABLE 2 Factors in Infectious Disease Emergence and Reemergence

Increased human intrusion into tropical forests
Lack of access to health care
Population growth and changes in demographics
Changes in human behaviors
Inadequate and deteriorating public health infrastructure
Misuse of antibiotics and other antimicrobial drugs
Microbial adaptation
Urbanization and crowding
Modern travel
Increased trade and expanded markets for imported foods

SOURCE: IOM, 1992.

Global Trade and Travel

Global trade has increased 1,000 percent since World War II. Sixty percent of global trade occurs in the Asia-Pacific region alone, resulting in an incredible movement of merchandise and people. Moreover, 20 percent of global agricultural trade occurs in Asia, which is the major destination market for U.S. trade goods, with the rate of agricultural product sales increasing 7 percent each year. As a large fraction of the economies of most developed nations are invested in trade, the level of exchange of goods will continue to increase.

One of the drawbacks to this movement of goods is that antimicrobial agents and other drug classes used to treat products may result in alterations in the ways in which people react to infections. Therefore, trade can introduce new pathogens or their vectors into a region through the shipping of contaminated products. In addition, increased world trade—combined with greater world travel—is precipitating some infectious disease events. Mitigation of these events requires greater investment in the public health infrastructure, disease investigation, sanitary infrastructure, strengthening of health ministries and other health agencies within governments, and coordinated action among the various sectors of society that deal with these issues.

Global travel also affects the transmission of infectious diseases. Nearly 1.5 billion travelers board airplanes every year, and the proportion of international arrivals among continents is increasing (Figure 5). The resulting effects include the importation of infectious diseases and infectious disease agents; for example, importation of influenza, pneumonic plague, TB, malaria, and even poliovirus by air travelers has been reported. In 1996, sporadic cases of yellow fever were diagnosed among travelers returning to the United States and Switzerland. Beyond tourism, as mentioned previously, migration also contributes to the spread of disease, which can be exacerbated when immigrants and refugees live in overcrowded and unsanitary conditions.

Seasonality and Climate Variation

The rise and fall in the rates of infectious diseases, particularly influenza, have long been associated with changes of seasons. In the tropical areas of the world there is a greater occurrence of influenza during the rainy season, and some believe that closer human contact during the rainy season in the tropics, when people tend to congregate indoors, might be responsible for more cases of influenza. This is in contrast to the epidemic situation in temperate regions, where there is a winter seasonality for influenza. In the winter, cooler, drier air favors the survival of influenza viruses, and just as in the tropics during the rainy season, people tend to congregate inside.

Other diseases show seasonal trends as well. Outbreaks of Venezuelan equine encephalitis in Colombia are associated with the rainy season. Respiratory syncytial virus (RSV) causes disease in the Northern Hemisphere in the

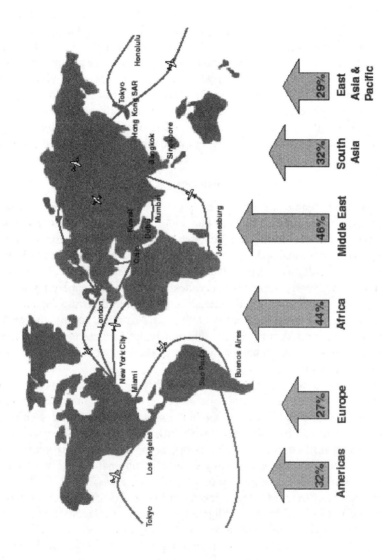

FIGURE 5 Frequent flyers: the most popular routes between continents, 1997. Percentage increase in international arrivals, 1993–1997. SOURCE: World Tourism Organization and Civil Aviation Organization.

winter and in the tropics during the rainy season. In England, for example, RSV is as important as influenza virus in causing morbidity and excess mortality among elderly people (Fleming and Cross, 1993).

The use of climate information for public health purposes deserves additional attention. Incorporation of climate and environmental variables into predictors of disease outbreaks could be an important tool for infectious disease prevention and control. For example, climate data have been used in retrospective analyses and modeling of Rift Valley fever outbreaks in East Africa. Refinement of such models could contribute to the planning for animal immunization programs. Knowledge and understanding of seasonal climate and meteorological conditions in West Africa have also been important for the elimination of onchocerciasis from that region. Historically, modeling has been used to predict malaria transmission on the basis of climate data, but the challenge to using these models is obtaining and validating quality data on the ground.

Zoonoses

In both developing and developed countries a number of new zoonoses (diseases transmitted from animals to humans) have emerged. These have been caused by either newly discovered pathogens or agents that are already known, often appearing in animal species in which the disease had not previously been detected. Zoonotic disease agents have also reemerged in some areas after being absent for many years, sometimes decades. Examples of emerging and re-emerging zoonotic disease agents include equine morbillivirus, Japanese encephalitis virus, and Australian bat lyssavirus in Australia, equine encephalitis virus in Colombia and Venezuela, enterohemorrhagic *Escherichia coli* in Japan, the bovine spongiform encephalopathy agent in the United Kingdom, and dengue virus in South America.

A dramatic example of a recent zoonotic disease outbreak was the occurrence of H5N1 influenza A virus—the so-called avian or bird flu—in Hong Kong in 1997 (Figure 6), which resulted in the slaughter of millions of chickens. Hong Kong is particularly vulnerable to infectious diseases because it is densely populated (6.68 million population in 1998), is in the crossroads between the East and the West, encounters a heavy volume of international travel, and has live poultry markets in close proximity to residential areas, which facilitate the spread of the virus from infected chickens to humans (see Chapter 4). Intense media attention to the outbreak highlighted the power of telecommunications to transmit images and mobilize and accelerate the response to an outbreak.

The juxtaposition of human and animal populations increases the likelihood of such outbreaks. Another example is Argentine hemorrhagic fever (AHF), which has been a major public health concern since 1955. The Argentine government is effectively using the AHF vaccine to reduce the incidence of disease. The incidence of AHF, however, has gradually increased among adult agricultural workers in rural areas, indicating an occupational exposure to the virus, and the focal incidence of AHF correlates well with the distribution of rodent infestation. The affected area in Argentina has gradually been extending and now covers approximately 150,000 square kilometers (58,000 square miles) including densely populated areas in parts of Argentina where the population at risk is approximately 5 million (see Chapter 2).

Of the novel zoonotic diseases, Hendra virus was first recognized as an outbreak of an unknown illness among horses in Brisbane, Australia. The virus was shown to occur naturally in fruit bats and to be widely distributed in northern and eastern Australia, as well as in Papua New Guinea. Hendra virus has been classified as the first member of a new genus in the family *Paramyxoviridae*. Studies of Hendra virus led to the discovery of Australian bat lyssavirus, a rabies-like virus, in both fruit and insectivorous bats. Australian bat lyssavirus is in the same group to which classical rabies belongs, antigenic group 1 of the lyssaviruses, but Australian bat lyssavirus can be differentiated from rabies virus on genetic grounds (see Chapter 4).

The emergence of zoonoses is likely to persist owing to increased human-to animal interactions, increased production and manufacture of animal-derived food products, changes in food-processing practices, and encroachment of human populations into feral animal habitats, as well as increased global trade and

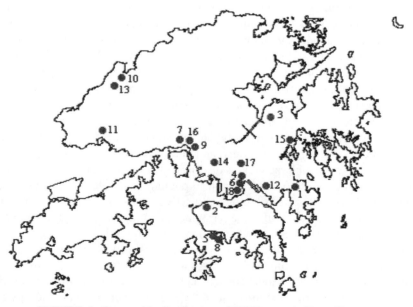

FIGURE 6 Geographic distribution of H5N1 cases in Hong Kong.

transportation of animals and animal products. Zoonotic outbreaks emphasize the importance of a robust public health infrastructure for disease surveillance and the need for international efforts and multidisciplinary collaboration to address such public health threats. Apart from human and animal health and welfare, due consideration must be given to the economic and political effects of zoonotic disease outbreaks.

Food Safety

Ensuring a safe food supply can have a large impact on the reduction of many common infectious diseases, such as diarrheal diseases, many of which originate in food products from animals. To reduce this impact, better, more reliable disease surveillance data are needed to effectively identify the cases of disease and to document the occurrence of specific pathogens and the sources of the infection. Much of the focus on food-borne disease control, however, is on other approaches, such as vaccines for animals raised for human consumption, and most of the public health community is not fully aware of the value of ensuring a safe food supply as a control mechanism.

Antimicrobial Drug Use in Animals and Humans

The use of antimicrobial agents in animal husbandry and agriculture is a mounting concern. In fact, about 50 percent of the antimicrobial agents produced are used in animal husbandry, agriculture, and horticulture. According to the U.S Department of Agriculture, during 1996 more than 136,000 kilograms (300,000 pounds) of streptomycin and oxytetracycline were sprayed on U.S. apples and pears to prevent or treat fire blight. In South Asia, rice fields and orchids are also sprayed with antibiotics to prevent blights and infections. These antimicrobial agents can enter the environment and then can enter humans through human ingestion of products contaminated with antimicrobicide residues.

The growth promoters and prophylactic antibiotics used in animal feed to promote health are subject to little regulation, however. In particular, fluoroquinolones are a valuable new class of drugs for use in humans. They are increasingly being used to promote health in poultry, from which the drug is excreted unchanged and remains biologically active after it is excreted, raising the potential for contamination of the environment and ingestion by other animals raised for human consumption. In fact, a publication from the state of Minnesota reported *Campylobacter* isolates from humans and as well as chicken in grocery stores that contained fluoroquinolone-resistant *Campylobacter*. Concerns about unrestrained practices are leading some Asian governments to control the animal feed being used on farms and to legislate the use of antibiotics and other drugs. In general, more efforts should be made to monitor isolates from food or food-source animals.

Equally troubling is the increase in the spread of drug-resistant microbes in humans (Table 3). Through the inappropriate use of antibiotics and normal microbial evolution, a growing number of infectious microorganisms are becoming drug resistant. For example, a resistant strain of the TB bacterium, *Mycobacterium tuberculosis*, recently appeared in the United States. Penicillin resistance has also been seen in strains of the microorganisms that cause pneumonia, meningitis, and middle-ear infections. In Argentina the rate of penicillin resistance among respiratory system pathogens, such as *Streptococcus pneumoniae* (24 percent) or *Haemophilus influenzae* (15 percent), is, on average, similar to that observed in Europe and the rest of the Americas; however, an alarming proportion of enteropathogenic isolates, like *Salmonella* and *Shigella* are resistant to first-line drugs. This phenomenon has not been observed in other regions. Hospitals worldwide are facing unprecedented crises from the rapid emergence of antibiotic-resistant microorganisms. Infectious diseases such as cholera, malaria, and tuberculosis—once thought to be nearly eradicated, particularly in developed countries—are making a comeback (Figure 7). In addition, the agents responsible for endemic and new diseases, including pneumonia and HIV/AIDS, are starting to develop drug resistance as well.

Drug-resistant forms of these diseases can become untreatable in any country. The impact of this trend could be reduced through better prescription practices, better training for health workers, better public education, and greater control over the availability of nonprescription drugs. National surveillance systems are needed to detect and respond to antimicrobial resistance in its early stages.

TABLE 3 Antibiotic-Resistant Disease-Causing Bacteria

Disease	Bacterium	Antibiotic Resistance
Dysentery	*Shigella dysenteriae*	Multidrug resistant
Gonorrhea	*Neisseria gonorrhoeae*	Penicillin and tetracycline resistant
Nosocomial infections:	*Enterococcus* species	Vancomycin resistant
	Klebsiella species	Multidrug resistant
	Pseudomonas species	Multidrug resistant
	Staphylococcus aureus	Methicillin resistant
Pneumonia	*Streptococcus pneumoniae*	Multidrug resistant
Typhoid	*Salmonella enterica*	Multidrug resistant

SOURCE: Workshop presentation by David Heymann, World Health Organization, 1999.

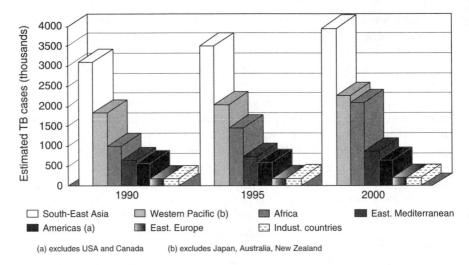

FIGURE 7 Tuberculosis in 1990, 1995, and 2000. There were 53,000 deaths/week in 1995. SOURCE: WHO/CDS.

Slowed Vaccine and Drug Development and Degraded Immunization Policies

More than 20 new infectious agents or diseases have been identified in the past 20 years, including toxic shock syndrome, HIV/AIDS, hantavirus pulmonary syndrome, and Nipah virus, to name just a few (Table 4). Like the organisms themselves, the challenges of detecting and preventing infectious diseases are constantly evolving. A strong, stable research and training infrastructure is needed to investigate the mechanisms of molecular evolution, drug resistance, and disease transmission to produce the knowledge that can lead to a vaccine or other effective means of preventing and treating an infectious disease. Just as an expanded research effort led to the discovery of protease inhibitors as treatments for HIV/AIDS, a renewed commitment to research is needed to ensure that similar successes are achieved for the numerous other infectious diseases currently threatening the earth's human population. Although vaccines against acute respiratory infections, diarrheal diseases, HIV/AIDS, malaria, TB, and dengue are desperately needed, vaccine development has lagged in the past 20 years. Vaccines are in the pipeline for Chagas' disease, onchocerciasis and lymphatic filariasis, leishmaniasis, schistosomiasis, and malaria, but these are in the predevelopment stage and still far from ready for use (WHO, 1999).

The rate of new antibiotic development has also slowed (Table 5). Industry is not always willing to invest in the development of a new class of antibiotics as readily as it was 20 or 30 years ago because of the financial risks involved. For

TABLE 4 Newly Identified Infectious Diseases and Pathogens

Year	Disease or Pathogen
1999	Nipah virus
1997	H5N1 (avian influenza A virus)
1996	New variant Creutzfelt-Jacob disease
	Australian bat lyssavirus
1995	Human herpesvirus 8 (Kaposi's sarcoma virus)
1994	Sabia virus
	Hendra virus
1993	Hantavirus pulmonary syndrome (Sin Nombre virus)
1992	*Vibrio cholerae* O139
1991	Guanarito virus
1989	Hepatitis C
1988	Hepatitis E
	Human herpesvirus 6
1983	HIV
1982	*Escherichia coli* O157:H7
	Lyme borreliosis
	Human T-lymphotropic virus type 2
1980	Human T-lymphotropic virus

SOURCE: Workshop presentation by David Heymann, World Health
Organization, 1999.

TABLE 5 Antibiotics Developed Since 1940

1940–1950	1951–1960	1961–1970	1971–1990	1991–1999
Bacitracin	Cycloserine	Gentamicin	Aztreonam	New versions of
Cephalosporin	Erythromycin	Lincomycin	Ciprofloxacin	Beta-lactams
Chloramphemicol	Fusidic acid	Nalidixic acid	Clindamycin	Quinolones
Framycetin	Kanamycin	Spectinomy-cin	Imipenem	Macrolides
Neomycin	Novobiocin	Tobramycin	Trimethoprim	
Penicillin	Rifampin			
Polymycin	Spiramycin			
Streptomycin	Vancomycin			
Sulfonamide				
Tetracycline				

SOURCE: Workshop presentation by David Heymann, World Health Organization,
1999.

example, the development of an antibiotic is an expensive process, and there is no guarantee that the antibiotic will remain effective before the patent period is over and the investment has been regained.

Globally, the number of individuals covered by immunizations, in addition to immunizations against polio, has risen since the advent of the global polio eradication initiative in 1990. However, standard immunizations for children are not as widespread as expected in many less developed regions of the world, where the risk of infectious diseases remains high. High vaccine costs, difficulties with administration (e.g., the logistics of refrigerating vaccines in tropical climates), and the number of vaccinations that each individual needs pose challenges to the implementation of more widespread immunization requirements, as well as posing challenges to immunization practices. In addition, when immunization programs are working well, they are sometimes forgotten. As a result, countries that have relaxed their immunization requirements are facing endemics and, in some cases, epidemics. For example, in Russia the pertussis vaccine component was dropped from the standard diphtheria-pertussis-tetanus vaccine preparation, resulting in an emergence of pertussis.

Another example is the risk of reemergence of poliomyelitis because of decreasing levels of vaccine coverage and indicators suggesting the breakdown of intensified surveillance, as currently seen in Haiti and the Dominican Republic. Although the last confirmed case of poliomyelitis on the North American continent was reported in June 1991, importation and spread of wild-type poliovirus strains into North America has been documented on two occasions in Canada (1992 and 1996), since then. The outbreaks occurred in members of religious communities that objected to and refused vaccination. This type of episode is especially problematic because of breakdowns in active surveillance.

Measles presents another example of how a disease that was nearly eradicated can be reestablished. Measles was on the verge of being controlled in Latin America in 1996, until the occurrence of outbreaks in Brazil, Argentina, and Bolivia. Now, Colombia and other countries in Latin America are in the final phases of the elimination of measles.

The need for basic immunization programs is often overshadowed by threats posed by new infectious agents with more dramatic clinical consequences. Although diseases like Ebola hemorrhagic fever receive much attention, diseases like measles do not. For example, in the Democratic Republic of Congo (formerly Zaire) in 1995, 350 people died from Ebola hemorrhagic fever in 1 year, whereas 350 children died from measles every 2 days. The challenge, in the words of a former director of the Centers for Disease Control and Prevention (CDC), William Foege, is to "link the fears of the rich with the needs of the poor." More intensive monitoring of immunization policies is needed to ensure that critical vaccinations are provided to the population. Those responsible for dissemination have to be reminded about the requirements of various vaccines, for example, that diphtheria-pertussis-tetanus vaccines should not be frozen.

NEED FOR COORDINATION AND COLLABORATION

Several governments have launched national efforts toward combating infectious diseases. In 1996 the United States announced new domestic and international surveillance and prevention efforts, including an initiative that seeks to improve research that will lead to new tools to detect and control emerging infectious diseases, as well as more basic research on the biology and pathology of infectious agents. The National Science and Technology Council's Committee on International Science, Engineering, and Technology Task Force on Emerging Infectious Diseases coordinated the overall initiative; the CDC and the U.S. Department of Defense (DOD) the surveillance and response efforts, and research activities were led by the National Institutes of Health. Threat reduction funds managed by both the U.S. Department of Defense and the U.S. Department of State are used to engage the former biological warfare facilities in the former Soviet Union in public health activities. The National Academy of Sciences has engaged in discussions with scientists at these facilities in collaborative pilot projects. For example, there is an attempt to reinvent the Stepnogorsk biological research facility in Kazakhstan, which previously weaponized the agent responsible for anthrax, to serve as a national TB reference center.

Other countries are developing and refining similar national plans. In Argentina, the objectives of a strategic plan to address emerging and reemerging infectious diseases include research and analysis of the results obtained by the country's diagnostic laboratories and application of the results of these analyses to surveillance and the development of policies related to infectious diseases. Since 1960, the Argentine National Epidemiological Surveillance System has collected information on 60 infectious diseases for which weekly notification by provincial public hospitals is mandatory. In addition, since 1992—after a cholera outbreak—the public health laboratory network for cholera has confirmed the results obtained through the mandatory notification process (see Chapter 2).

Mexico has instituted special surveillance programs in response to natural disasters. After such events, for example Hurricane Mitch, new infectious disease events are exacerbated by the migration of individuals from Central America into Mexico, as well as the hygienic problems caused by the heavy rainfall and flooding. A program in five Mexican states performs the laboratory diagnosis of dengue, leptospirosis, enterobacterial infection, and cholera. The program also provides reagents to laboratories and performs quality control testing and training (see Chapter 2) (Figure 8).

The United Kingdom has developed a pandemic influenza contingency plan. It defines the roles and responsibilities of all the organizations and people who would be involved in the response to a new pandemic. The plan moves in phases from the interpandemic period, to an outbreak outside the United Kingdom, to outbreaks within the United Kingdom, to the pandemic stage and the end of the pandemic. Currently, the effort is to bring the plan into concordance with that of WHO (see Chapter 5).

Other efforts have been explicitly transnational. For example, a project developed jointly by the African Regional Office of WHO, the CDC, and the U.S. Agency for International Development (USAID) aims to improve the well-being of the approximately 600 million people currently residing in the 47 member states of the African Regional Office of WHO. The project implements integrated infectious disease surveillance and improved epidemic preparedness and response (see Chapter 3).

Correspondingly, in June 1995 the Pan American Health Organization (PAHO) convened a meeting of international experts to discuss strategies for the prevention and control of emerging infectious diseases. As a result of that meeting, a regional plan of action was prepared to develop regional and subregional approaches and to guide member states in addressing specific problems (Figure 9). The regional plan has four goals: (1) strengthening regional surveillance networks for infectious diseases in the Americas; (2) establishing national and regional infrastructures for early warning about and rapid response to infectious disease threats through multidisciplinary training programs and enhancement of laboratory capabilities; (3) promoting the further development of applied research in the areas of diagnosis, epidemiology, prevention, and clinical studies; and (4) strengthening the regional capacity for effective implementation of prevention and control strategies (see Chapter 2).

The European Union (EU) has changed the environment for public health issues in Europe by providing funds and the opportunity to share information.

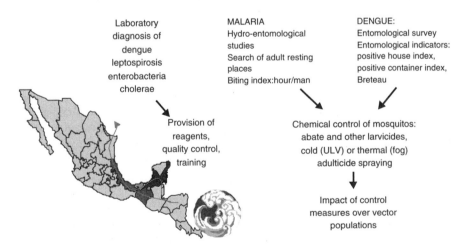

FIGURE 8 Surveillance in response to natural disaster. "Operativo Frontero Sur" XII/98–III/99: Campeche, Chiapas, Quintana Roo, Tabasco and Veracruz. SOURCE: INDRE.

Although that part of the world does not face the same types of infectious disease problems found in Asia and Latin America, it has a unique set of infectious disease issues with which it must contend. For example, in Sarajevo, Bosnia-Herzegovina, and other parts of Eastern Europe in 1993–1994, WHO had to establish new communicable disease surveillance because of anxieties about the re-emergence of some diseases, in particular, typhus, diphtheria, and TB (see Chapter 5).

The capacity to enhance communicable disease control efforts in Europe was further advanced by the Delphi technique for consensus building. Data information and exchange that provide an earlier warning and detect infectious disease threats that require international coordinated action were identified and evaluated at the national levels. Questionnaires and feedback rounds circulated among a group of experts from individual European countries were among the data collection methods used. The results of the Delphi exercise were submitted to the European Commission (EC) as part of its expert advice to EC members on the development of communicable disease surveillance at the European level. Influenza was ranked among the high-priority diseases requiring international surveillance.

DOD is establishing a syndromic surveillance system called the Early Warning Outbreak Recognition System, in Indonesia. Once every 24 hours several sites around the Indonesian archipelago report data on clinical syndromes to a central point in Jakarta, where a DOD laboratory is collocated with the Indonesian Ministry of Health. The system is conducted out of hospitals located around Indonesia, where nurses collect syndromic data from patients. These data are entered into a database into which one can enter not only the signs and symptoms but also the specific working diagnosis. In close to real time the frequencies of various syndromes can be tracked across the Indonesian archipelago.

Emerging infections require substantial multisectoral and multinational approaches, as well as sufficient funds. Additional examples of collaborative efforts and the various mechanisms by which they can be achieved are described below.

Cooperation Across Borders

Nations that share borders are sometimes the most logical place to initiate efforts. For example, the CDC Division of Quarantine is collaborating with Mexico on a pilot sentinel surveillance project along the U.S.-Mexico border for febrile exanthemas and hepatitis. This effort aims to strengthen the sensitivity of infectious disease surveillance through the observation of clinical syndromes and to enhance the public health capacity along the border through surveillance efforts at the provider level. A binational notification process informs the appropriate officials in each country of any reported infections. The protocol calls for rapid local, regional, and national sharing of information about sentinel cases of

20

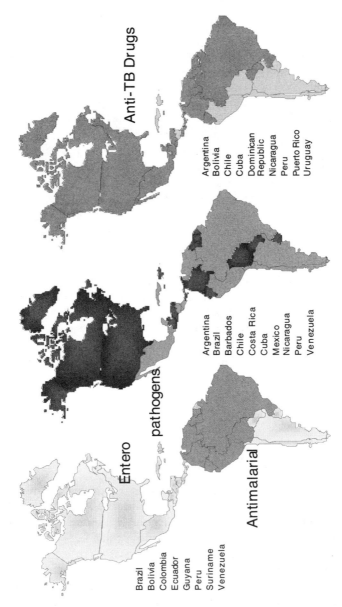

FIGURE 9 Regional CD surveillance. Countries participating in drug resistance surveillance. SOURCE: PAHO/WHO.

illness or disease that meet either country's notification requirements. Similarly, Brazil and Argentina are investing in strengthening a network of laboratories.

The trend toward globalization of public health is not without its problems. Some countries believe that these efforts undermine their ability to protect the health of their citizens or to retain state sovereignty. Some countries are concerned about the diminishment of their authority within their own territories. This can be especially contentious among bordering countries. Thus, international and national laws, regulations, and practices must be understood and discussed in the context of establishing cooperative efforts. Local needs must be recognized and addressed.

Bilateral Agreements

In recent years the U.S. and South African governments have discussed the issues of AIDS and TB at key bilateral and multilateral meetings. Similarly, in bilateral meetings with Russia, the United States has raised awareness of TB and promoted the use of directly observed treatment (short course), an inexpensive strategy for the detection and treatment of TB. Emerging infectious diseases have also been discussed under the Asian-Pacific Economic Cooperation (APEC), as well through the U.S.-European Union New Transatlantic Agenda. Discussions surrounding debt relief at trade summits have identified the health care system as a priority for infrastructure development in the poorest countries.

Bilateral and multilateral trade agreements signed between Argentina and its neighboring countries (Bolivia, Brazil, Chile, Paraguay, and Uruguay) have included health protection components. Since the 1970s, emphasis has been given to health of the populations within the borders of each country, and internationally agreed upon health care and safety standards (see Chapter 2).

International Health Regulations

In 1969, the International Health Regulations aimed to ensure maximum security against the international spread of diseases with minimum interference with world trade, tourism, and business. The regulations set out a series of guidelines for monitoring and surveying the normal ports of a vector's entry into countries (airports, seaports) so that agents that might arrive on conveyances do not spread from the port area. The regulations require reporting of a relatively small number of infectious diseases: yellow fever, cholera, and plague. There are disincentives to reporting, which diminish the value of the program. For example, when cholera has been reported, some countries have erected economically damaging trade barriers around the country that reported cholera. Furthermore, reporting does not always result in a response.

New regulations are being drafted that will cover more infectious diseases and that will require electronic communication among quarantine officers. Ef-

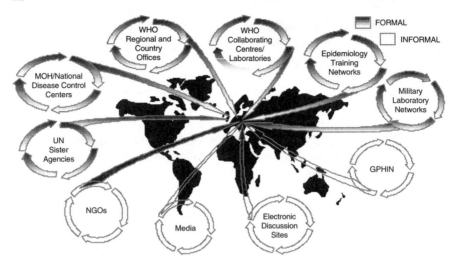

FIGURE 10 Global surveillance of communicable diseases: a network of networks.
SOURCE: WHO/CDS.

forts are being made to increase the response capabilities of all countries and to decrease the stigma of reporting. Critical aspects of international collaboration are establishing trust and harmonizing epidemiological and laboratory practices. Conflicts can arise around jurisdictions, costs, and international politics. Furthermore, countries have different traditions in terms of accountability and data dissemination that must be acknowledged. In addition, conflicts among international agencies and with nongovernmental organizations (NGOs) will inevitably occur. The potential for disagreement must be recognized and dealt with early in the course of an infectious disease outbreak.

NETWORKS OF GLOBAL SURVEILLANCE

Current global surveillance comprises a network of networks (Figure 10), as well as electronic discussion sites and the media. Some of these are laboratory networks, others are epidemiology training networks, and still others are reporting networks. Between November 1996 and June 1998, 260 outbreaks were reported through these networks. Once they are validated, reports of the outbreaks are distributed to a limited number of health professionals to improve the level of awareness of reported outbreaks that might have international implications. The new international health regulations may require that some actions be taken against countries that are not reporting.

Global Epidemic Intelligence, established by WHO in 1996, was created to improve international preparedness for epidemics by sharing the same information in a timely fashion, thereby countering confusing information that may be disseminated. Confusion can have a major impact on the international prevalence of a disease. Through active collection of information about ongoing outbreaks worldwide, including validation of the sources of information and the rapid verification of the outbreak, WHO is able to share this information with those who need to know. The Internet provides an unprecedented opportunity for information sharing.

Efforts are under way to establish networks for the surveillance of emerging infectious diseases in nine countries of the Amazon Region and the Southern Cone Region. A plan of action was developed for each region in collaboration with international reference centers, including CDC, the University of Texas Medical Branch at Galveston, and the U.S. Army Medical Research Institute of Infectious Diseases. The network should be able to perform active surveillance on the basis of a syndromic approach. Five disease syndromes were selected for both regions, and two additional ones were recommended for the Southern Cone Region. The five syndromes are undifferentiated febrile syndrome, hemorrhagic fever, febrile icteric syndrome, acute respiratory distress syndrome, and sudden unexplained death.

The WHO Global Influenza Surveillance Program, now 50 years old, was responsible for the early identification of the H5N1 influenza A virus, as well as the H9N2 virus that occurred later. The program has served as a model for many surveillance programs established in subsequent years. It is an action-oriented program. Because WHO must issue recommendations for the composition of influenza vaccines twice a year—once for the Northern Hemisphere in February and once for the Southern Hemisphere in September—data must be gathered throughout the year. The infrastructure in place allows the identification of new variants, whether they are new epidemic variants or new variants with pandemic potential. The infrastructure rests on a number of national influenza centers that serve as the key laboratories for the isolation and identification of influenza viruses, using a kit of reagents produced by CDC and distributed globally. The laboratories also collect epidemiological information for transmittal to WHO headquarters in Geneva. International collaborating centers conduct comparative analyses of influenza viruses from all over the world. Collaboration with industry is essential because the strains that are identified as vaccine candidates are provided free of charge to the pharmaceutical industry for vaccine production.

In September 1998, the European Parliament and the Council of Europe agreed to establish a network for the epidemiological surveillance and control of communicable diseases in the community. This effort, which became active in July 1999, builds on an established set of networks for individual diseases such as travel-related Legionnaire's disease, HIV/AIDS, and TB, networks for drug resistance surveillance and the EntreNet for enteric organisms. National surveillance institutes have collaborated in looking at standards for surveillance. A field epidemiology training program, European Programme for Intervention Epidemiology Training, trains people in the science of epidemiology and establishes communication among public health authorities from different countries. Regular surveillance bulletins in both paper and electronic form have been produced. In addition, inventories of capacity and capabilities across Europe have been generated, including a directory of vaccination policies.

Despite these multiple national and international efforts, existing and planned networks focus on known infectious diseases, which means that new agents may go undetected. A future challenge will be to transform established methods and infrastructures to detect and respond to known diseases and novel infectious agents. DNA sequence-based analysis, polymerase chain reaction-based analysis, and multicomponent-array chips will increasingly allow rapid identification of stray nonhuman DNA that is present in internal organs or blood. Deployment of these technologies will require money and awareness.

Continuing Need for Local Surveillance

Even with extensive intranational and cross-national cooperation, local surveillance remains the most important function in the early warning of and response to infectious diseases. At the local level, disease intelligence functions enhance the ability to assess indicator events. Individuals in charge of surveillance systems at the local level must work closely with their colleagues in the agricultural and veterinary sciences and those who are conducting disease surveillance in related fields. These systems must also adapt to changing patterns of health care, for example, the trend toward patients calling nurses for assistance rather than visiting a general practitioner's office, where surveillance data might be collected. Local efforts need to be integrated so that local, national, and international efforts are not competing or being duplicated. Databases must be interrelated and designed so that they can be linked while protecting confidentiality and privacy.

Local efforts also reveal much about behavioral change measures that might be required. For example, revised guidelines for dengue control elevate behavioral change indicators to the same level as entomological or epidemiological indicators, using as a model behavioral surveillance for HIV/AIDS. This requires more bottom-up surveillance programs, modeled after many nutrition and child health programs, in which indicators can be used at the household level; for example, households can determine whether removing domestic containers that may be sources of mosquito breeding is either improving the dengue situation or making the dengue situation worse. This is an important approach, as it paves the way for consumer-based control measures for other diseases, such as the use of insecticide-treated mosquito nets or the use of domestic aerosols for the control of malaria in Africa.

NGOs can play a progressive role in this area by being proximate to the problem and, through advocacy, ensure that infectious disease control issues are placed on local, national, and international agendas. NGOs can develop pilot programs, conduct assessments, provide training, and contribute to the wider implementation of surveillance and control efforts. Accordingly, NGOs must have access to affordable and essential drugs and must have sustained financing to support long-term intervention activities and programs.

Preservation of Samples

The availability of archived biological samples can facilitate understanding of new pathogens and can speed the response to outbreaks. Therefore, more countries must be encouraged to preserve blood and tissue specimens, whether from zoonotic or human events, to make it feasible to search for specific susceptibility factors. For example, an outbreak of viral encephalitis caused by the previously unrecognized Nipah virus occurred in Malaysia in 1998. The ability to analyze archival collections of serum samples from pigs collected in Malaysia in 1995 showed that some porcine samples had antibodies to Nipah virus. This allowed investigators to conclude that the virus had been circulating in the population for some time.

A large and invaluable resource of archived samples is DOD's triservice serum repository, begun in 1985, which contains 25 million specimens collected from military personnel. This resource serves many research needs; it most recently provided important information on hantavirus from samples obtained from military recruits from the southwest United States.

Using the Internet for Reporting and Communication

The Internet is providing a whole new means for the posting of disease alerts and information about new therapies and technologies, informing public health officials about relevant meetings, and providing new opportunities for collaboration. The Internet is increasingly being used as a source of outbreak-related information through media newswires, electronic discussion groups, and websites. Quality assurance, however, is an important requirement for officials using worldwide web-based information as a source of infectious disease information.

To explore the extent to which this form of nontraditional reporting can be channeled for good use, WHO developed with the Canadian Ministry of Health a computer application that scans thousands of websites 10 times a day, including media newswires, for information that could lead to a report or reports of communicable diseases or disasters. This information is then transmitted to WHO. The Global Public Health Intelligence Network serves as an example of an innovative new approach to surveillance. Of about 450 outbreaks verified in the past 2.5 years, more than 50 percent of the reports came from the media. "Hits" gathered from websites are then monitored to obtain more detailed information. This information is entered into a database that also contains data from more traditional reporting mechanisms.

TAKING ADVANTAGE OF
WINDOWS OF OPPORTUNITY

Too often, delayed responses to outbreaks and the spread of infectious diseases result in missed opportunities for treatment and control. Lessons from the past should teach people today about the dangers of missing important openings for intervention. For example, in Africa the rates of resistance patterns to penicillin and tetracycline by the organism that causes gonorrhea are on the rise. In the 1950s and 1960s, when the prevalence of gonorrhea throughout African countries was extremely high governments did not attempt to change behavior or offer treatment. Had public health education been offered back in the 1960s and had antibiotics been used effectively, gonorrhea would not be present to the same extent throughout Africa today and would not be causing needless suffering and infertility in women. Today, HIV poses a similar new challenge, as several African countries have infection rates of greater than 25 percent. Many believe that the opportunity to halt the spread of this deadly virus has already been missed.

Fighting the global spread of infectious disease takes political resolve and sufficient financial resources, just as eradication of smallpox did. In many cases, the tools required to detect, isolate, and control microbial agents are available but are underused or inaccessible. For example, measles vaccination rates in Africa range from 19 to 90 percent. A vaccine exists for hepatitis B and *Haemophilus influenzae* type B infection, yet the perception of the burdens of these diseases relative to those of other diseases and the costs of vaccines against both pathogens has led to their low level of use. The health system required to deliver these vaccines needs to be strengthened. In addition, government policies that can lead to the censuring of information about the extent to which a disease such as HIV/AIDS is present in the population undermine disease surveillance and control activities.

Some parts of the world are ripe for intervention. For example, there is an enormous need and opportunity to introduce new infectious disease control infrastructures into the Central Asia republics and Russia because their relatively new state of independence has left them with no experience in international procurement and self-governance. For example, they lack the logistical wherewithal to purchase reagents or vaccines or implement directly observed therapy. USAID, CDC, the Soros Foundation, and WHO have been collaborating to bring the necessary resources to these evolving health care systems.

The eradication of smallpox, which was declared in 1980, serves as an example of an effective worldwide effort to engender political will and muster resources. The disease, which was causing as many as 1.9 million deaths a year by the late 1960s, was eradicated because of concerted efforts to further develop an effective vaccine and to create a global infrastructure for its distribution and for smallpox surveillance. Today, the use of linkages through the Internet offers several possibilities for faster reporting and faster responses to disease threats. It must be recognized, however, that even the fundamental tools needed to capitalize on new information technologies may not be available in some of the developing countries, and training workshops are needed when new tools are introduced.

Although many developing countries are aiming for self-sufficiency in developing, storing, and maintaining necessary supplies of reagents and in-country expertise, organizations such as CDC, WHO (including PAHO and other regional offices), USAID, and NGOs will be needed to supply routine diagnostic reagents, provide training, enhance communication, and exert quality control. More structured agreements are needed to ensure that the requisite laboratories are adequately equipped and that channels of communication are left open.

A structured agreement that could bring technology transfers, communication, and reporting into a coordinated program to strengthen public health laboratories and surveillance is the Biological Weapons Convention. Article X of the Convention requires that the signatories exchange technologies. This would improve the diagnostic capabilities of laboratories and improve information sharing. These enhanced capabilities could also add to those resources used to support the public health capabilities of laboratories in other countries. Similarly, the medical research laboratories of overseas military assets can help local civilian medical communities find ways to adapt the many new and emerging detection technologies to infectious disease surveillance. Training and education activities sponsored by the military could also be coordinated with those programs administered by the public health infrastructures of governments and NGOs.

To achieve an integrated system of surveillance and monitoring with an appropriate and timely response, the world community must work toward the following common goals:

- Strengthening disease surveillance of humans and domestic animals. Priority areas include improving communication and information sharing between the medical and veterinary communities and designing integrated medical and veterinary disease surveillance systems at the regional level.
- Building on existing disease-specific reporting systems. Consider the use of novel technology, such as remotely sensed data, in existing disease surveillance systems and expand disease-specific surveillance systems to monitor other closely related diseases.
- Enhancing and improving the use of communication and information technologies.
- Promoting the International Health Regulations.
- Developing improved, low-cost laboratory infrastructure for surveillance.

- Fostering good public health practices.
- Training personnel.
- Educating the public and professionals to slow the rate of increase of antimicrobial resistance.
- Conducting collaborative research. Priority areas for investigation include preventing the development of drug-resistant microbes by promoting the appropriate use of antibiotics; understanding the transmission patterns of food-, water-, vector-, and air-borne pathogens; and improving diagnostic tests and prevention and control strategies for infectious diseases.
- Accelerating vaccine development and distribution.
- Fostering credible coordinating international groups.
- Encouraging overseas institutions, such as military medical research units, to be more involved in helping the host country develop an infectious disease surveillance infrastructure.

All nations should promote the participation of the health sector in international trade agreements that may affect human, animal, or plant health. This requires a commitment at the highest levels of government to improve the components of the global surveillance system, upgrading the infrastructure and the qualifications of the human resources needed to control emerging infections, and supporting and encouraging rapid intra- and intercountry communications on health issues, including infectious disease outbreaks. This kind of high-level dialogue must be intentional and ongoing. Outreach to countries not involved in international discussions on disease surveillance is especially important, as they are most likely at high risk for infectious disease outbreaks. Within and across borders there must be integration of the public health system, epidemiologically, building on the laboratory and the clinical health care base. This requires efforts at the local level.

Economic globalization, demographic changes, and the increased costs of infectious disease control and prevention for human health and welfare emphasize the interdependence of all nations. As efforts are made to improve trade and bring democratic governance to countries in the developing world, the crucial needs of public health cannot be forgotten. Strengthened national and regional public health systems not only will reduce the level of human suffering from infectious diseases but also can promote economic growth and political stability among those countries most affected.

Introduction

David Heymann, M.D., M.T.M.
Executive Director, Communicable Diseases
World Health Organization, Geneva

LOST WINDOWS OF OPPORTUNITY

Emerging infectious diseases are closing, or have the potential to close windows of opportunity for infectious disease eradication or elimination. The 20th anniversary of the eradication of smallpox provides a reminder of an opportunity of which the world took advantage. Smallpox had been a devastating disease with high transmission and case-fatality rates. In 1969 alone, smallpox caused 1.6 million deaths. The eradication of smallpox stands as one of the outstanding achievements in the history of public health. Eradication was achieved because of a worldwide effort that was supported by the necessary political will and human and technical resources. The world took advantage of opportunity for smallpox eradication because a safe vaccine was available.

In the year that smallpox was declared eradicated, human immunodeficiency virus, HIV, appeared and rapidly colonized Africa and the world. Today, the prevalence of HIV is greater than 25 percent in some adult populations, such as in the Democratic Republic of Congo (formerly Zaire). In the United States, a military recruit who was immunized against smallpox developed generalized vaccinia because he was HIV seropositive, and died. That tragic event highlights the fact that if the global smallpox eradication campaign had been postponed, the world would not have been able to eradicate smallpox as easily as it did before 1980.

Many other opportunities have been lost. In the 1950s and 1960s, gonorrhea was highly prevalent throughout African countries. Governments did not attempt to change behavior to prevent transmission. Treatment either was not offered or was infrequently offered. When available, treatment for sexually transmitted diseases was many times more expensive than treatment for other diseases, especially in the private mission hospitals throughout Africa. Therefore, gonorrhea largely went untreated and disease prevalence increased to a less manageable level. Today, gonorrhea is present throughout Africa, where it causes infertility in women and where it is one of the major driving forces in the HIV epidemic, facilitating the transmission of HIV. Had effective public health education been in place in the 1960s to help change sexual behavior and had antibiotic treatment been used effectively, there would not be such a great problem with gonorrhea today. In this case, a window of opportunity to control one disease and reduce the rate of transmission and impact of a far more serious disease has closed.

The prevalence of tuberculosis (TB) and multidrug-resistant TB is increasing globally. The emergence of HIV facilitated the resurgence of TB, which provides another example of a case in which an opportunity has been lost. Global surveys show that there is a 1 percent prevalence of resistance to at least one TB drug. Multidrug treatment for TB costs between $20 and $30 for a complete cure, but treatment costs are approximately $3,000 for multidrug-resistant TB. In many places, the chance to achieve a manageable level of TB by the proper use of drugs has been lost.

The global effort in the 1960s and 1970s to eradicate malaria succeeded in eradicating malariologists, but not malaria. Today, the malaria parasite is resistant to the drugs of choice—chloroquine or pyrimethamine-sulfadoxine (fansidar), or both—because of improper treatment. Drug-resistant malaria takes longer to respond to treatment. In addition, the mosquito species that transmit the parasite are resistant to the insecticide that previously controlled them because of the improper use of insecticides and a breakdown of public health infrastructure. A window of opportunity to eliminate malaria and mitigate its impact has been lost as increasing numbers of adults are losing work and more children are dying because of the resurgence of malaria.

Many public health opportunities have also been lost because of the emergence of infectious diseases. Poor public health practices by the local hospital workers in Kikwit, Zaire, drove the 1995 Ebola hemorrhagic fever outbreak. A cycle of transmission among the patient care staff transmitted the virus to their families and additional patients. The international community learned of the outbreak in May 1995, nearly 20 weeks after the first case was reported. Poor communication, poor infection control practices, and poor preventive public health measures reflect the weak public heath care systems and the poor state of infectious disease surveillance in most of Africa. With the end of the Cold War, the end of the colonial era, and the decline of Western interest in tropical diseases, the public health infrastructure in many African countries has deteriorated. Infectious disease surveillance is nearly nonexistent, and emerging infections frequently go unreported.

Immunization, the vanguard of public health practice, is losing ground in both developing and developed countries. For example, the rate of immunization against yellow fever is declining in most countries of the world, particularly those countries where the yellow fever virus is endemic. It is very difficult to have an African government commit to programs of vaccination against yellow fever as part of routine immunization programs, even though the vaccine is safe and inexpensive and engenders long-lasting immunity. In addition, tourists are becoming less and less rigorous in their vaccinations. Recently, there was an international alert when a photographer returned to Germany with an unknown disease. At first it was thought to be Ebola hemorrhagic fever, but yellow fever was confirmed to be the diagnosis.

Climate variability and climate change are closing other windows of opportunity as the distribution of some diseases is expanding as a result of changing climatic conditions. The traditional meningitis belt ran across Saharan Africa. Recently, epidemics have occurred farther south in the countries of Uganda, Kenya, and Tanzania. The spread of meningitis may be due to the extreme droughts brought about by changing climate conditions in those areas.

The bovine spongiform encephalopathy (BSE) outbreak in cows in the United Kingdom, with the subsequent resulting outbreak among humans of a variant of Crcutzfcldt-Jacob disease (vCJD), is an example of carelessness in food-handling practices and public health measures. That is, in the late 1970s the procedures for rendering bonemeal and other products from animal carcasses changed. The resultant food products were used in animal feed. However, infectious agents were transmitted through the animal feed from infected carcasses back into ruminants, resulting in the BSE epidemic and the transmission of the BSE agent to humans, resulting in vCJD.

At a time when infectious diseases are on the rise—when 48 percent of deaths between birth to 44 years of age are largely due to one of six infectious diseases and when in the span of 20 years AIDS has become the second most important infectious killer in the world—the costs of treating infectious diseases are also rising. At the same time, infectious diseases are taxing economies. The 1991 cholera epidemic in Peru cost that country an estimated $770 million. The plague epidemic in India cost that country $1.8 billion. Between 1990 and 1998, BSE in the United Kingdom is thought to have cost more than $6 billion. Although, while these diseases may not be high on the list of causes of mortality, they are high on the list of causes of economic morbidity.

GLOBAL RESPONSES TO EMERGING INFECTIONS

Among the global responses used to combat emerging infections are the International Health Regulations (IHR). The World Health Organization (WHO) administers the IHR. The purpose of the IHR is to ensure maximum security against the international spread of diseases with minimum interference in world traffic (travel and trade). The IHR ascribe a set of norms at ports of entry into countries so that diseases or their vectors, which might arrive on conveyances, do not spread beyond those port areas. At the same time, they require the reporting to WHO of any occurrence of one of three diseases: cholera, yellow fever, and plague. The IHR are limited in that they require reporting of only those three infectious diseases, even though many more infectious diseases are of equal or greater threat to human health and healthy economies. Consequently, the IHR are being revised to cover more infectious diseases and will be directed out of WHO headquarters in Geneva, Switzerland, using electronic communications for quarantine officers. The revised IHR also seek to increase the capability to report disease outbreaks and to decrease the stigma of reporting, as frequently there is a disincentive to reporting because other countries may respond by erecting trade barriers against the reporting country, such as those against countries that have reported cholera epidemics. The IHR will likely play a larger role in the future global surveillance and control of infectious diseases.

Two tools are used globally to control infectious diseases: eradication and elimination. *Eradication* is an important activity that has been used successfully in the past against smallpox. Current efforts to eradicate polio are nearing completion. In addition, by the end of 2001 or early 2002 it is anticipated that wild-type poliovirus transmission will be interrupted worldwide. *Elimination* is decreasing the prevalence of a disease to a level at which it can be more easily handled within the health care system. Lymphatic filariasis is a disease with a low mortality rate but with a high rate of morbidity and severe negative effects on local and regional economies and social structures. Efforts toward the elimination of lymphatic filariasis are under way in Africa following the guaranteed donations in perpetuity by Merck & Co. and SmithKline Beecham of the drugs necessary to control the disease. In an attempt to take advantage of the powerful partnership with the private sector, other efforts are under way to eliminate leprosy and Guinea-worm infection (dracunculiasis).

Elimination and eradication programs need a strong global surveillance system. These systems may be either formal or informal networks; both are equally important and serve a valuable role. The formal networks, such as laboratory networks, epidemiology training networks, and other groups, are networking and continuously reporting on diseases. Informal networks are often electronic discussion sites, such as ProMed and the Global Public Health Intelligence Network of Health in Canada (GPHIN). The news media, nongovernmental organizations, the Red Cross, and Doctors Without Borders (Médecins sans Frontières) are also among the many informal networks. WHO monitors the surveillance networks and validates suspected outbreaks of disease, sharing news of disease outbreaks with the global health community. Through this program, WHO identified about 215 infectious disease outbreaks between November 1996 and June 1998.

WINDOWS OF OPPORTUNITY FOR THE FUTURE

Strengthening global surveillance is not enough to eliminate or eradicate infectious diseases. Laboratories need strengthening and an improved means of communications and reporting. Networks of laboratories that link countries and regions need to be established so that appropriate actions include those people who can help the most. One means of strengthening laboratories is to work closely with those monitoring the Biological Weapons Convention. Article X of the Convention requires the signatories to exchange technologies. This effort would bring technology transfers into a coordinated program that would strengthen those signatories' laboratories. This effort would also add to those resources that support laboratories in other countries, for few donors are interested in strengthening laboratory capacity.

Most donors are more likely to fund the "glamorous" disease control programs. However, basic public health laboratories are not strengthened. To assist with that effort to strengthen basic public health laboratories, the Center for Disease Control and Prevention is helping support diagnostic testing for meningitis and other laboratory capabilities. The U.S. Agency for International Development is also taking interest in surveillance and strengthening of laboratories.

In the future, closer ties between public health and trade organizations will be needed. Recent discussions between WHO and the World Trade Organization are exploring ways in which WHO would become an arbiter in certain trade issues with a public health component, especially in the case of infectious diseases, through IHR. Closer links are also needed in the area of food safety and IHR.

Greater collaboration is also needed between the medical and behavioral science communities. Changes in human behavior have been effective in controlling the spread of HIV in Thailand and Uganda. Yet, only those two countries have had success in this area. More time needs to be spent investigating the behavioral determinants and interventions needed for effective disease control.

The world as a whole is not putting enough effort into research and development of new vaccines. Despite several outbreaks caused by the Ebola and Marburg viruses, the global community has never been able to put together a solid research effort to discover the origins and natural histories of these viruses. Most of the investigations have been conducted with whatever funds are available at the end of a fiscal year.

Emerging infections are also requiring multisectoral approaches. For example, the world cannot address the growing problem of antimicrobial resistance among microorganisms that cause disease in humans in isolation from other sectors of society that are also involved. The fields of animal husbandry, agriculture, medicine, and public health need to work together through advocacy and public health awareness campaigns.

Creative ways are needed to secure adequate funding for infectious disease research, surveillance, and prevention programs in both the private and the public sectors. Currently, about 10 percent of health research worldwide is directed toward the needs of developing countries by both the public and the private sectors, but only 2 percent of that money is going toward the six most important infectious disease processes in those countries: AIDS, malaria, respiratory infections, diarrhea, TB, and measles. The directions of both public- and private-sector research need to be refocused back toward infectious diseases.

Emerging infections are a critical phenomenon. The globalization occurring in the world community provides a reminder of this fact. Efforts to combat emerging infections require a global response to provide adequate financial support. Public commitment needs to be developed, for where there is public commitment it will be followed by political resolve, and where there is both political and public determination there are windows of opportunity to eradicate and eliminate infectious diseases.

2

Emerging Infections in Latin America

OVERVIEW

Economic globalization, demographic change, and the rapidly rising costs of health care in all countries are converging factors that transcend national borders. In Latin America, economic globalization has meant the increased movement of people and goods and changes in environmental and occupational health hazards—often occurring in the context of political instability. It has also meant that health risks are being transferred. For example, an epidemiologic transition, marked by a gradual increase in the rate of noncommunicable diseases, is now under way in the region. In the next 25 years it is expected that the dominant diseases in Latin America will increasingly become like those of the United States and other more industrialized nations, where depression, heart disease, and cancer are the primary health problems. The infectious etiologies of chronic conditions will be of increasing importance and will require action. Thus, the opportunities for the transmission of emerging and reemerging infectious diseases remain and in some instances have increased. As the region's needs change, the responses of national and international health agencies are evolving. Cooperative actions and solutions for infectious disease surveillance and response among government health agencies and between countries are key elements needed to address the common problems of emerging infections in Latin America.

EMERGING INFECTIONS IN COLOMBIA:
A NATIONAL PERSPECTIVE

Jorge Boshell-Samper, M.D.

Director General, Instituto Nacional de SaludBogotá, Colombia

Several key elements are responsible for the resurgence of infectious diseases in Colombia, including: environmental changes; human demographics, mosquito behavior, and deforestation; emerging antimicrobial resistance; political decentralization and complacency; and natural disasters. Although tuberculosis (TB) is considered a major emerging disease in the developed world, it has always been prevalent in Colombia and does not fit the criteria and concepts of an emerging infection. It has been a continuous threat.

Environmental Changes

Unpredictable and unusually heavy rainfalls have resulted in the emergence of Venezuelan equine encephalomyelitis (VEE) virus outbreaks that afflicted thousands of horses and humans in Colombia and Venezuela. Although the disease had been silent for more than 20 years, outbreaks occurred in 1992, 1995, and 1998. The immediate response involved vaccination of horses with the TC83 vaccine. An international research project that involved a collaboration between the University of Texas Medical Branch at Galveston, the Instituto Nacional de Higiene of Venezuela, and the Instituto Nacional de Salud (INS) of Colombia was launched to understand the epidemiology of enzootic sylvatic disease cycles and their mechanisms of emergence as epizootic strains that killed horses. In addition, increased surveillance of VEE virus-infected horses was conducted through a national laboratory-based network system.

Seasonal rainfall changes were also associated with the reemergence of influenza epidemics that afflicted hundreds of individuals throughout the country: influenza A/Wuhan/H3N2 in 1996, influenza B/Beijing and influenza A/Sydney/H3N2 in 1997, influenza A/Sydney/H3N2 in 1998, and influenza A/pending/H3N2 in 1999. The Colombian response was the implementation of a regular sentinel surveillance system sponsored by INS for influenza and other respiratory viruses. This surveillance system will be for prediction of and planning for the next influenza pandemic in the region. The information obtained from the surveillance system underscores the importance of research.

Human Demographics, Mosquito Behavior, and Deforestation

Dengue was a forgotten disease in Colombia by the 1950s and 1960s because of the eradication of *Aedes aegypti*, the mosquito vector. After reinvasion, of the country by *Ae. aegypti* the country experienced multiple epidemics. In the

1970s the four serotypes of dengue virus were documented and in the 1980s dengue virus serotypes 1, 2, and 4 infected thousands of patients. Because *Ae. aegypti* spread horizontally throughout lowland areas of the country and also spread vertically up the populated cordilleras, a series of parallel mountain ranges, dengue fever is now endemic and causes frequent epidemic peaks. Moreover, dengue hemorrhagic fever (DHF) has emerged as an epidemic illness, with 39 registered cases in 1990, followed by 100 cases in 1991 and 359 cases in 1992. The incidence of DHF per 100,000 population in Colombia rose from 0.11 in 1990 to 9.82 in 1997.

Colombia has responded with an aggressive medical and public health education program in medical schools and with local and regional symposia with public health providers and local and foreign scientists as speakers (sponsored by the Pan American Health Organization (PAHO) or the Colombian Ministry of Health). In addition, the country adopted community-based education programs, educated the public through national television programs, and adopted municipality-based biological control programs. It also made sporadic attempts at mosquito control. The real goal is to implement a strategy to develop a dengue vaccine through cooperation between INS and the Instituto de Immunologia, Universidad Nacional de Colombia.

In the American region enzootic for yellow fever, Colombia is the only country that has escaped jungle yellow fever (JYF) outbreaks for more than 10 years, despite serious and constant civil unrest and intense illegal activities in the jungles of Colombia. However, the emergence of urban yellow fever remains a Sword of Damocles for the country, because most isolated cases of JYF, among patients still in the viremic phase of their infection, are found in hospitals located in urban centers full of *Ae. aegypti*, the urban vector of yellow fever virus (Breteau indexes [see the glossary in Appendix A], over 60 percent). The response has been to update the 17D yellow fever vaccine manufacturing plant to implement good manufacturing practices and implement a stringent program for the detection and diagnosis of febrile cases of yellow fever among individuals in the jungle of the Amazon and Orinoco regions.

An outbreak of acute Chagas disease myocarditis was diagnosed for the first time in Colombia during April and May 1999 in a rural municipality on the Caribbean coast. The best hypothesis to explain this epidemic implicates ecological changes brought about when the palm trees in the neighborhood were cut down. An increased surveillance program has been initiated.

Emerging Antimicrobial Resistance

Clones of *Streptococcus pneumoniae* with diminished susceptibility to penicillin (DSP) or with multidrug resistance are emerging in Colombia, as documented by the PAHO/SIREVA project. From 1994 to 1996 the rate of DSP was low (12 percent), but the rate of resistance increased yearly and by 1997 it had reached 39 percent, along with the emergence of multidrug-resistant (clones 23F and 14B). Furthermore, 42.4 percent of the DSP population studied was found to be multidrug resistant. The Colombian response has been to continue the national surveillance program with the Colombian Pneumococcal Study Group and public health programs to detect changes in the susceptibility pattern.

The annual parasitic index (API which is the number of parasitologically confirmed cases per 1,000 population per year) for malaria has continuously increased in Colombia from 1970 (API = 1) through the end of the 1990s (API = 6). This increase is due to a variety of factors, including resistance to antimalarials (resistance to chloroquine in *Plasmodium falciparum* was first reported in 1961), vector resistance to pesticides, and the breakdown of public health measures. There has been major support for the development and improvement of a synthetic antimalarial vaccine (SPf66), primarily by Manuel E. Patarroyo at the Instituto de Immunologia, Universidad Nacional de Colombia. Furthermore, multicenter studies have been conducted in areas of malaria endemicity to develop community-based programs for vector control.

Complacency and Natural Disasters

Despite the elimination of poliomyelitis in the Americas, there is a risk of the reemergence of this disease through importation, decreasing levels of vaccine coverage, and breakdown of intensified surveillance, as currently seen in Haiti and the Dominican Republic. Although the last confirmed case of wild-type derived poliomyelitis on the North American continent was reported in June 1991, the risk of importation and spread of wild-type poliovirus strains into the Americas has been documented on two occasions in Canada (1992 and 1996). This type of episode is especially problematic because of breakdowns in active surveillance and decreased vaccine coverage.

Colombia and the rest of Latin America are in the final phases of measles eradication. After measles was on the verge of control in 1996, outbreaks in Brazil, Argentina, and Bolivia are reminders of the reality of the reestablishment of transmission. Decentralization of health services in the process of health reform requires that national surveillance and control be conducted through INS, a step being implemented by the Colombia Ministry of Health.

Public health authorities are very much aware of potential disease outbreaks after natural disasters. Active surveillance after the earthquakes in Armenia and the coffee-growing region of Colombia brought attention to the fact that an apparent outbreak of hepatitis A had been endemic and undiscovered for more than 3 months before the disaster. In addition, an urban malaria outbreak was diagnosed for the first time in more than 30 years.

Conclusion

The constantly changing and unpredictable factors that contribute to the resurgence of infectious diseases in Colombia require increased and sustained surveillance.

A NATIONAL STRATEGY FOR EMERGING INFECTIOUS DISEASES: THE ARGENTINE CASE OF 1999

Elsa L. Segura, Ph.D.

Director, Administración Nacional de Laboratorios e Institutos de Salud
"Dr. Carlos G. Malbrán" (ANLIS MALBRAN), Ministry of Health
Buenos Aires, Argentina

Emerging infectious diseases have increasingly been detected in Argentina, starting with epidemic outbreaks of Argentine hemorrhagic fever (AHF) in the 1950s, human immunodeficiency virus infection (HIV)/AIDS and leishmaniasis in the 1980s, and cholera, antimicrobial resistance (e.g., resistance of meningococcus type B and *Mycobacterium tuberculosis*), hantavirus, and dengue in the 1990s.

Argentina has a population of 36 million and comprises a federal organization of 23 provincial states and the city of Buenos Aires. The national health system is coordinated at the political and technical levels by the Federal Health Council (COFESA), which meets at least six times a year. At the central level, the Directorate of Epidemiology is in charge of national epidemiological surveillance. Laboratory responsibilities are led by the Administración Nacional de Laboratorios e Institutos de Salud "Dr. Carlos G. Malbrán" (ANLIS MALBRAN), a decentralized national administration that coordinates 11 health institutes and centers and a network of 650 laboratories distributed throughout the country, with a presence in each one of the provincial states. Networked activities include research and development, training, production of biologicals, and quality control for the diagnosis of diseases affecting public health. In recent years there has been enhanced cooperation of these networks with the epidemiological efforts of the Argentine Ministry of Health.

External quality control was enacted in 78 percent of the network laboratories in 1999. As a direct result of these efforts, the laboratories cooperated in writing national guidelines for diseases subject to mandatory notification.

The objectives of the strategic plan of ANLIS MALBRAN for emerging and reemerging infectious diseases are research and analysis of the results obtained by the diagnostic laboratories and application of these analyses to surveillance and policy development. Since 1960 the Argentine National Epidemiological Surveillance System (enacted by law) each week has collected information on 60 infectious diseases for which notification by provincial public hospitals is mandatory, making its findings available to the public. Since 1992—after a cholera outbreak—the public health laboratory network for cholera has confirmed the results obtained through the mandatory notification process.

At present, the surveillance system in Argentina includes three components: (1) physicians at the first health care level (sentinels), (2) public health laboratories distributed throughout the country, and (3) provincial epidemiology units that analyze the collected data. Applied research and quality assurance processes—directed to increasing the specificity of epidemiological surveillance—occupy a central role in the organization of the 650 laboratories in the Argentine network.

Argentine Hemorrhagic Fever

Argentine hemorrhagic fever (AHF) has been a major public health concern since 1955. It is an acute viral disease caused by the Junin virus, an arenavirus, and it is endemic to the Argentine humid pampa. An increased incidence of AHF has been observed among adult rural workers, reflecting occupational exposure to the virus. The focal incidence of AHF correlates well with the distribution of the rodent reservoirs. The affected area has gradually been extending and now covers approximately 150,000 square kilometers (58,000 square miles), including densely populated areas in the Department Rosario in the province of Santa Fe. The population at risk is approximately 5 million. AHF has shown 5-year cycles, likely related to fluctuations in the densities of rodent populations.

Because the control of rodent reservoirs of the Junin virus is not feasible in such an extended geographical area, most preventive efforts have been directed to vaccine development. The development of a vaccine against AHF has a long history. In a first stage (1968–1969), a live, attenuated, cloned virus vaccine, XJ Clon 3, was developed in the Faculty of Medicine at the University of Buenos Aires (Weissenbacher et al., 1969) and was tested successfully in 300 volunteers. In a second stage, a clone from the Junin virus formed the Candid 1 vaccine, developed as a result of an international cooperative project between the U.S. Army Medical Research Institute of Infectious Diseases (USAMRIID), PAHO, and the Argentine Ministry of Health. Between 1985 and 1990 a vaccine trial involving more than 7,000 volunteers in Argentina established the immunogenicity, inoculability, and efficacy (95.5 percent) of the Candid 1 vaccine.

The vaccine was readily accepted by the population, which was significant considering that vaccination was voluntary, experimental, restricted geographically, required an informed consent as well as a pregnancy blood test for women of reproductive age, and required travel to designated vaccination posts, which were open only on certain fixed days at fixed times (Enria et al., 1998).

The Candid 1 vaccine is highly effective; it elicits high levels of protective antibodies for 9 years after vaccination in approximately 90 percent of people vaccinated with a single dose. However, AHF is not an eradicable disease, and despite good vaccine coverage rates, isolated cases and limited outbreaks will likely occur in the future. Therefore surveillance aimed at detection and prompt treatment of people with AHF and research on the activity of the Junin virus in the rodent reservoirs must remain active. Research on AHF and development of an effective vaccine demonstrated that a developing country can solve its own infectious disease problems and enhance an initiative through international cooperation.

HIV/AIDS

The cumulative number of HIV/AIDS cases in Argentina was 15,166 as of July 31, 1999. Because of a delay in the notification process, however, approximately 17,000 cases may have occurred up to that date (Ministry of Health and Social Welfare of Argentina, 1999). Surveillance is carried out through mandatory notification, and only laboratory-confirmed cases are reported. The system uses the reporting criteria of the Centers for Disease Control and Prevention except for the determination of CD4/CD8 cell counts.

Leishmaniasis

An epidemic of cutaneous-mucocutaneous leishmaniasis occurred in the province of Salta in northwestern Argentina between 1984 and 1987. The etiologic agent was identified as *Leishmania (Viannia) braziliensis.* The local incidence rate rose from 6.4 cases per 100,000 in 1984 to 28.7 cases per 100,000 in 1985 (Sosa Estani et al., 1998). Since October 1997 there has been an increase in the number of cases in the departments of Orán and San Martín (Salta), close to the site of the upsurge from 1984 to 1987, whereas other outbreaks were detected in the northeastern province of Misiones. The rising incidence rate was likely associated with traditional deforestation activities in Salta and climatic phenomena in Misiones.

Cholera Epidemic

The first case of cholera was reported in Argentina in the summer of 1992 and was caused by *Vibrio cholerae* O1 biotype El Tor, serotype Ogawa, producer of the cholera enterotoxin (CT). The epidemic started in the northwestern province of Salta, and spread to neighboring areas in the provinces of Formosa and Jujuy. Sporadic cases occurred later in other areas after the movement of the population from the affected areas (Varela, 1994). By June 1995, four epidemic outbreaks had occurred, mainly during the summer months. National health authorities determined that only bacteriologically confirmed cases of cholera would be reported in the country. As a consequence, hospital laboratories performed an essential role in diagnosing cases of cholera. Contrary to the serotype prevalent in the rest of the Latin American region, Ogawa was the most prevalent serotype (91.8 percent) in Argentina, and 99.2 percent of the isolates produced CT, as determined by enzyme-linked immunosorbent assay (ELISA). During the second and third outbreaks, only 24 (1.7 percent) isolates presented with resistance to antibiotics. Among these isolates, seven were resistant to tetracycline. In addition, five isolates presented with unusual multidrug resistance, accompanied by β-lactamase activity against broad-spectrum (third-generation) cephalosporins.

Hemolytic-Uremic Syndrome

Hemolytic-uremic syndrome (HUS) is an endemic disease that affects children younger than 5 years but that most frequently affects children between the ages of 6 and 36 months. Cases mainly occur during the warm season and include eutrophic children, children with good nutrition, and those living under good hygienic conditions. In many of the affected infants, the diarrhea that occurs during the prodromal period is the first diarrhea of their lifetimes.

Reporting of HUS was made mandatory in 1999. Age- and gender-specific incidence and prevalence rates are estimated according to data reported by hospital-based centers of nephrology to the Nephrology Commission of the Argentine Pediatric Society. In 1998, the total number of reported cases was 227. The incidence rate was 6.8 per 100,000 children younger than 5 years, with a 2 percent mortality rate. More than 6,000 cases have been reported in Argentina since 1963. The central and southern provinces have the highest incidence rates. The mortality rate decreased from 15 percent in 1965 to 2 percent in 1998 as a consequence of early specific diagnosis, knowledge of disease physiopathology, and therapeutic measures, such as the implementation of peritoneal dialysis for severe forms of HUS with oliguria and anuria (Rivas et al., 1994).

Bacterial Antibiotic Resistance

In Argentina the rate of penicillin resistance of respiratory system pathogens, such as *Streptococcus pneumoniae* (24 percent) and *Haemophilus influenzae* (15 percent), is, on average, similar to that observed in Europe and other countries in the Americas. However, for some enteropathogens, like *Salmonella* or *Shigella*, an alarming proportion of isolates are resistant to first-line drugs. This phenomenon has not been observed in other regions.

Outbreaks of nosocomial infections of multidrug-resistant *Salmonella* have been reported for more than 7 years, particularly in hospitals located along the northeastern rivers in the provinces of Buenos Aires, Entre Rios, Corrientes, Santa Fe, and Misiones. All isolates produce an extended spectrum β-lactamase and the CTX-M2, as well as aminoglycoside acetyltransferase AAC(3)II and AAC(6)I enzymes which inactivate aminoglycosides. The corresponding genes are located in a conjugate plasmid of high molecular weight. These resistant genes were also detected in *Vibrio cholerae* isolates during the second and sixth cholera outbreaks.

In general, in Argentina the proportions of gram-negative bacilli resistant to β-lactam antibiotics (40 to 60 percent), aminoglycosides (4 to 32 percent), or trimethoprim-sulfamethoxazole (45 to 62 percent) are three times higher than those observed in developed countries (Rossi et al., 1999).

The new cephalosporins and aminoglycosides are first-line drugs for the treatment of severe infections. The most efficient resistance mechanism involves the production of extended-spectrum β-lactamase-inactivating enzymes and enzymes that modify aminoglycosides. In Argentina a national reference laboratory (Rossi et al., 1999) is in charge of coordinating the network of 200 countrywide laboratories and is part of the World Health Organization (WHO) international program of antimicrobial resistance surveillance (WHONET). It is necessary, therefore, to provide training on standardized methods for sensitivity studies, design quality control programs for microbiological diagnosis, and to develop national reference laboratories to verify, characterize, and be alert to the development of new resistance mechanisms.

Multidrug Tuberculosis Resistance

The Argentine National Tuberculosis Control Program reported 12,205 cases of TB in 1998 (400 cases fewer than in 1997). The decrease in the number of reported cases reflected a 5 percent reduction in the morbidity rate, from 35.5 per 100,000 population in 1997 to 33.8 per 100,000 population in 1998. The incidence of TB decreased by 18 percent relative to that in 1993. In 1998, the program was notified by 1,700 fewer cases than the number in 1993. The case notification rate in Argentina was 33.9 per 100,000 in 1998.

All 650 laboratories of the TB diagnostic network use bacilloscopy. Isolation through culture is performed in approximately 100 laboratories; 18 perform sensitivity tests and identification by biochemical tests. Two national laboratories characterize isolates by biochemical procedures and hybridization.

The National Tuberculosis Control Program surveys the magnitude and characteristics of *Mycobacterium tuberculosis* resistance to antibiotics; the last trial was conducted in 1994. Initial resistance trends for TB unrelated to AIDS have not changed since 1968. However, acquired resistance trends have increased, especially in recent years, because of multidrug resistance (simultaneous resistance to at least isoniazid and rifampcin). Nevertheless, resistance levels are not yet alarming. Furthermore, to improve cure rates and block the transmission chain, the rate of directly observed therapy (short course) was 95 percent in 1999, whereas it was 74 percent in 1996.

In Argentina, a close relationship has been observed between multidrug-resistant TB outbreaks, HIV infection, and hospitalization in infectious disease hospitals located in big cities (e.g., Buenos Aires and Rosario). However, a serious increase in the rate of multidrug-resistant TB was also observed in patients without evidence of HIV infection who had a history of TB treatment.

Hantavirus Pulmonary Syndrome

Hemorrhagic fever with renal distress (HFRS), geographically restricted to Asia and Europe, was until 1993 the only disease known to be caused by hantaviruses. In 1993, a new clinical entity emerged in the United States—hantavirus pulmonary syndrome (HPS)—characterized by severe acute respiratory distress. Its etiologic agent was identified as a new hantavirus, Sin Nombre virus. HPS is a viral zoonosis transmitted to humans by inhalation of the excreta of infected rodents.

In Argentina, infection of wild and laboratory rodents as well as subclinical human infections were reported between 1983 and 1985. Clinical cases presenting as both HFRS and HPS were retrospectively diagnosed between 1987 and 1996.

In March 1995, the first case of a familial outbreak of HPS was reported in El Bolsón, in southern Argentina. As of December 15, 1996, a total of 77 cases of HPS has been reported (with a 48 percent fatality rate) in the southern, northern, and central regions of Argentina. During this outbreak, data suggested for the first time the possibility of person-to-person transmission (Enria et al., 1996, Wells et al., 1997). A retrospective case-control study carried out to identify risk factors associated with HPS showed that people who have had physical contact with an HPS patient or his or her bodily fluids and who shared a room with a patient with HPS were at increased risk of acquiring the disease. Person-to-person transmission was evaluated by comparing the viral sequence homologies of viruses from 16 epidemiologically linked patients with HPS (nosocomial or household contacts) (Padula et al., 1998). As of November 1999, 255 accumulated cases of HPS had occurred in Argentina.

Dengue

Several cases of dengue were reported in northern Argentina between 1905 and 1911. In 1916, an outbreak of 15,000 clinically diagnosed cases was reported in eastern Argentina. In 1955, the vector mosquito *Aedes aegypti* covered 15 million square kilometers (5.8 million square miles), reaching the city of Buenos Aires. By 1963, *Ae. aegypti* was considered eradicated, but 12 cases of dengue were confirmed between April and October 1997, the first occurrence since 1916.

At present, *Ae. aegypti* occupies the same distribution range as it did in 1955—including the city of Buenos Aires—according to data collected by the

Table 2-1 Health Component of Bilateral Trade Agreements, Argentina, 1980–1999

Health Agreement	Argentine Law Number, Date	Subject	Protocol
Bolivia-Argentina (ARBOL)	22.253, July 16,1980	Transmissible diseases in border zone, epidemic outbreaks	Cholera, malaria, Chagas' disease, dengue, hemorrhagic fever
Paraguay-Argentina	23.435, July 28, 1986	Transmissible diseases in border zone	Same as ARBOL plus health control of migrant population
Uruguay-Argentina	24.116, August 5, 1992	Transmissible diseases in border zone, medical technology	Same as ARBOL, plus HIV/AIDS, emerging infectious diseases, joint epidemiological surveillance
Paraguay-Argentina	24.836, July 27, 1996	Transmissible diseases in border zone, nutrition, environmental engineering, local development	Joint surveillance in border zone, emerging infections, Chagas' disease
Chile-Argentina	25.130, August 4, 1999	Promotion, protection, exchange of technology, health in border zone	Information about emerging infections in border zones, network of scientific and technical information

SOURCE: Oscar González Carrizo, Dirección de Relaciones Internacionales, MSAS, Argentina.

Argentine Ministry of Health. In preparation for the future, the Ministry of Health is strengthening entomological actions through community-based control programs. Laboratories are building a network for the diagnosis of dengue infections by MAC ELISA. In 1998, a dengue outbreak occurred in the province of Salta (Aviles et al., 1999). In total, 644 cases of dengue (58 percent, affecting 10 localities between January 3 and May 31, 1998) were detected by laboratory-based diagnostic methods. Dengue serotype 2 virus was isolated and was implicated in the outbreak. Clinically, all cases corresponded to classical dengue. This is the first time that a dengue outbreak was diagnosed by laboratory-based means in Argentina and also the first time that dengue virus was isolated in the country.

Bilateral and Multilateral Agreements

Bilateral and multilateral (Mercosur) trade agreements signed between Argentina and neighboring countries (Bolivia, Brazil, Chile, Paraguay, and Uruguay) have included a health protection component (Table 2-1). Since the 1970s, emphasis has been given to health in the borders zones and internationally agreed upon quality and safety standards.

The goal is to promote the participation of the health sector in international trade agreements that may affect human, animal, or plant health from an early stage of the negotiation process. Current objectives are: (1) improve the three components of the surveillance system, especially the efficacy of surveillance at sites distant from the most populated districts, including the border zones; (2) upgrade the infrastructure and qualification of human resources; and (3) permit rapid intra- and inter-country communications on health issues, including outbreaks.

DIAGNOSIS, EPIDEMIOLOGICAL SURVEILLANCE, AND CONTROL PROGRAMS FOR EMERGING AND RE-EMERGING INFECTIOUS DISEASES IN MEXICO

Ana Flisser, D.Sc.[*]
Director, Instituto Nacional de Diagnóstico y Referencia Epidemiológicos (INDRE) Secretaria de Salud (SSA), Colonia Santo Tomas, Mexico

Transitions in disease epidemiology are the result of the social transformation of a developing country such as Mexico and the forces that give rise to new health risks. These risks include both nontransmissible diseases and transmissible diseases. However, it is the spectrum of transmissible diseases that is changing rapidly in conjunction with changes in society and the environment. These diseases are considered either emerging or reemerging infections, and epidemiological and laboratory surveillance for these types of infections are at the center of Mexico's disease control efforts. For this purpose, the Secretary of Health (SSA) in Mexico has established a Coordination of Epidemiological Surveillance activity through the National Institute of Epidemiological Diagnosis and Reference (INDRE), the National Public Health Laboratory, the Directorate of Epidemiology, and several disease control programs. This section presents the

---

[*]The author gratefully acknowledges the personnel from the National Institute of Epidemiological Diagnosis and Reference, the National Network of Public Health Laboratories, the Coordination of Epidemiological Surveillance, the Directorate of Epidemiology, and the AIDS National Council for the information provided in preparing the manuscript. Special thanks are given to Alejandro Escobar for critical comments on the manuscript.

current state of surveillance for the most important emerging and reemerging infectious diseases in Mexico.

Dengue

Dengue has become an epidemiological priority in Mexico, and the etiological detection of dengue virus is mandatory. Figure 2-1 shows the number of samples that INDRE has analyzed for dengue in the last 4 years. The rate of positivity for dengue virus-specific antibody has been approximately 40 percent in all years, suggesting that clinicians have an adequate case definition of dengue, especially since dengue symptomatology can be pleomorphic. As shown in Figure 2-1, the number of samples analyzed by INDRE has decreased because samples are increasingly also processed by the National Network of Public Health Laboratories (NNPHL). However, reference procedures for dengue virus serotype identification performed by cell culture or polymerase chain reaction (PCR) are performed only at INDRE. These specialized assays have detected an important increase in serotype 3 dengue virus (Figure 2-2), suggesting that the Mexican population is susceptible to this virus serotype. PCR is performed preferentially for hemorrhagic cases to provide the result in less than 48 hours. Many samples submitted for viral identification from patients with suspected dengue virus infection are negative. These may be false-negative results because of the short period of time during which virions can be detected in serum and also the presence of other, not considered, etiologies of the disease. During 1996 and 1997, analysis by PCR gave higher rates of positivity than the rates obtained by cell culture, whereas during 1997 and 1998 the two assays had similar rates of positivity. Early on, only samples from patients with well-characterized hemorrhagic cases of dengue virus infection were subjected to PCR to ensure adequate performance of the technique. Later on, samples from patients with a less stringent definition of dengue virus infection were accepted for stronger support of the infectious epidemiology.

Leptospirosis

Leptospirosis has been documented in Mexico for more than 20 years, according to serological studies. Evaluation for leptospirosis is the first option in the differential diagnosis of dengue. In 1998, 8 percent of samples negative for dengue virus had antibodies to *Leptospira*. Different serological variants (serovars) are associated with exposure to different animals. For example, abattoir workers who handle pigs are more likely to have antibodies to the *pomona* serovar, whereas dog owners have antibodies to the *canicol* serovar.

Tuberculosis

In contrast to dengue, the incidence of TB in Mexico is stable, although multidrug-resistant *Mycobacterium tuberculosis* strains are emerging. Laboratory studies for the diagnosis of TB are performed in 637 laboratories belonging to the NNPHL. An evaluation of these laboratories revealed that the microscopes in one-third of the laboratories were in need of repair, one-quarter of the laboratories did not have sufficient reagents, and across the laboratories half the personnel needed training. Of the 32 states that make up the Republic of Mexico, 7 do not have the proper facilites and equipment (e.g., safety cabinets or centrifuges with aerosol containment lids) to culture mycobacteria. In response to the laboratory inspection, microscopes were repaired and more than 350 microscopists attended INDRE for a 3-day update course. In addition, laboratories acquired the needed reagents and, in collaboration with the Centers for Disease Control and Prevention (CDC), conducted proficiency tests for external quality control. Also in collaboration with CDC, a *M. tuberculosis* drug resistance study conducted in three states shows that the proportion of isolates with acquired resistance to isoniazid and rifampin is within the expected limits (22.4 percent), but the proportion of isolates with primary resistance is very high (2.4 percent for both drugs). After improved laboratory quality control and surveillance, it was found that 61 percent of TB cases are located in 160 municipalities. A directly observed supervised therapy program has recently been organized in these municipalities.

HIV/AIDS

Since 1996, the number of new cases of HIV/AIDS has peaked at about 4,000 per year in Mexico. The prevalence is highest among homosexual and bisexual men, male sex workers, and intravenous drug users. The prevalence has decreased remarkably among those who receive blood transfusions. Coordinated efforts have been made in recent years to distribute reliable screening kits for antibody detection to blood banks and NNPHL. In addition, intensive information and education campaigns are under way, including a recently published edition for clinicians that contains guidelines on the diagnosis, management, and treatment of patients with HIV/AIDS. Specialized medical services for patient management were recently established in most Mexican states. An independent component of the SSA, called FONSIDA, has been established to provide antiretroviral treatment for infected persons who cannot afford it through specialized medical services. FONSIDA began by treating children and pregnant women and has recently included other groups of adults. INDRE and the National Institute of Nutrition are responsible for performing tests to determine viral load and have standardized the assays for viral load determination.

Other Emerging and Reemerging Diseases

Cholera reemerged in Mexico in 1991 and was characterized by a steep increase in the number of cases, reaching 16,430 cases in 1995. The incidence of cholera has markedly declined since then, and few cases are now reported. This may be a consequence of the intensive control measures that have been implemented, but the precise reason for the impressive reduction in the number of cases of cholera is not known. Rotavirus infection has been detected more frequently in children younger than 3 years, mainly in the winter. The most common serotypes circulating are Gl, G2 and G3, P1, and P2, with mixtures of serotypes being found. Chagas' disease (the causative agent for which is *Trypanosoma cruzi*), previously considered rare in Mexico, has been associated with blood transfusion, with rates of occurrence above 1.4 percent in some states. It is now mandatory for blood banks throughout Mexico to search for antibodies to *T. cruzi,* in addition to antibodies to HIV and hepatitis viruses, in blood from donors.

Studies performed in Mexico and elsewhere have shown that an individual infected with the intestinal adult tapeworm (*Taenia solium*) is the main risk factor for neurocysticercosis among household occupants. This disease has been a public health problem for many years in developing countries and is now considered an emerging infectious disease in some developed countries such as the United States. With the aid of modern diagnostic assays and by asking patients if tapeworm segments are seen in feces or if there are cases of late-onset epilepsy in the family, it is possible to identify tapeworm carriers and provide them with successful treatment. This approach is being tested in two political jurisdictions of two Mexican states (a population of more than one million) by educating all physicians who provide primary care in health centers through social service activities.

Surveillance in Response to Natural Disasters

Mexico has instituted a special surveillance program in response to natural disasters. In recent years, earthquakes and extreme climate events, such as heavy rainfalls, hurricanes, and flooding in several states, have created the need to establish field laboratory facilities in affected communities for the diagnosis of dengue, leptospirosis, enterobacterial infection, and cholera. The program also provides reagents, training, and quality control activities. In 1998 this surveillance program analyzed more than 38,000 blood, fecal and environmental samples from seven states for leptospirosis, dengue, malaria, cholera, and enterobacteria. The prevalences of the first three diseases by laboratory diagnosis were 14, 5, and 3 percent, respectively. Among the 6,859 fecal samples collected, 87 were positive, 3 contained *Vibrio cholerae* O1, 24 contained *V. cholerae* non-O1, 5 contained *Salmonella*, 1 contained *Shigella,* and 54 harbored *Escherichia coli*. Of 8,642 environmental samples assayed, 380 contained *V. cholerae* non-O1.

After natural disasters, large-scale entomological studies on the malaria and dengue vectors are performed before and after chemical control efforts. These studies help define the impact that the control measures have on the mosquito populations and disease transmission. The results from those studies are used to support disease control decision making by field health brigades that remain in the disaster areas as long as they are needed. Seven thousand localities with approximately 850,000 homes were surveyed in 1999, and more than 600,000 medical appointments were provided.

In summary, SSA has made an intensive effort to diagnose, survey, and control emerging and reemerging diseases in Mexico. It is hoped that other countries can learn from the Mexican experience with combating the threats from emerging and reemerging infections in their efforts to help better understand these diseases and to prevent and mitigate their impacts.

RESPONSE OF THE PAN AMERICAN HEALTH ORGANIZATION TO COMBATING EMERGING INFECTIOUS DISEASES IN LATIN AMERICA AND THE CARIBBEAN

Francisco Pinheiro, M.D.
Advisor on Viral Diseases, Program for Communicable Diseases
Pan American Health Organization, Washington, D.C.

In the Americas, a complex array of factors has contributed to the recognition of an increasing number of emerging, and reemerging infectious diseases. The problem is marked by the appearance of new pathogens causing disease of marked severity, such as HIV, arenaviruses, and hantaviruses. Simultaneously, old pathogens—such as those that cause cholera, plague, dengue hemorrhagic fever, and yellow fever—have reemerged and are having a considerable impact in the Americas. Microorganism mutations that lead to drug-resistant and multi-drug-resistant strains of *Mycobacterium tuberculosis*, enterobacteria, staphylococci, pneumococci, malarial parasites, and other agents have been occurring and are becoming major obstacles to the control of these infections.

In response to this alarming trend, in June 1995 PAHO convened a meeting of international experts to discuss strategies for the prevention and control of emerging infectious diseases. As a result of this meeting, a regional plan of action was prepared to develop regional and subregional approaches and to guide member states in addressing specific problems. The regional plan has four goals: (1) strengthening regional surveillance networks for infectious diseases in the Americas; (2) establishing national and regional infrastructures to provide an early warning of and a rapid response to infectious disease threats through multidisciplinary training programs and laboratory enhancement; (3) promoting the further development of applied research in the areas of diagnosis, epidemiology, prevention, and clinical studies; and (4) strengthening the regional capacity for effective implementation of prevention and control strategies.

Subsequently, PAHO has implemented activities in accordance with the regional plan, taking into consideration priorities that have been reviewed since 1996 on an annual basis by PAHO's Task Force on Surveillance for Emerging and Reemerging Diseases.

Efforts are under way to establish networks for the surveillance of emerging infectious diseases in nine countries of the Amazon Region and the Southern Cone Region. A plan of action was developed for each region in collaboration with international reference centers, including CDC, the University of Texas Medical Branch at Galveston, and the U.S. Army Medical Research Institute of Infectious Diseases. The network should be able to perform active surveillance on the basis of a syndromic approach. Five disease syndromes were selected for both regions, and two additional ones were recommended for the Southern Cone Region. The five syndromes are undifferentiated febrile syndrome, hemorrhagic fever, febrile icteric syndrome, acute respiratory distress syndrome, and sudden unexplained death.

In view of growing evidence of an alarming increase in the rate of antimicrobial drug resistance in the Americas and other parts of the world, strengthening of surveillance of the antimicrobial resistance of selected enteropathogens, mainly to monitor the patterns of resistance of salmonellae, shigellae, and *Vibrio cholerae*, has been implemented for the past 3 years in 15 countries of Latin America and the Caribbean in collaboration with the Laboratory Centers for Disease Control in Canada. The goals of this project include strengthening diarrheal disease surveillance, improving national laboratory capabilities, standardizing methodologies for diagnosis, establishing a network of national reference laboratories, and creating databases of emerging antibiotic-resistant organisms.

Since 1996, five workshops have been conducted on subjects such as laboratory and epidemiology relationships, diagnostic methods, antiserum production, data analysis, proficiency testing, and external quality assurance. In addition, a project addressing the basis for the prevention and control of antibiotic resistance in the Americas has been proposed by PAHO. The objectives of this project are (1) to decrease the incidence and spread of antimicrobial resistance and, consequently, improve the treatment of infectious diseases, and (2) to provide for more effective delivery of interventions for the control and prevention of antimicrobial resistance. A project to strengthen a regional system for epidemiological surveillance is under way. The PAHO strategy used to achieve this has been to focus on (1) improved national surveillance, (2) the development of a regional electronic platform to collect and communicate surveillance data, (3) training in outbreak detection and response, and (4) surveillance of antimicrobial resistance. Several activities are being implemented, including training workshops to improve the system.

3

Emerging Infections in Africa

OVERVIEW

As a region, Africa is characterized by the greatest infectious disease burden and, overall, the weakest public health infrastructure among all regions in the world. Frequently, vertically oriented disease surveillance programs at the national level and above in Africa often result in too much paperwork, too many different instructions, different terminologies, too many administrators, and conflicting priorities. Streamlined communications, strengthened public health surveillance, the use of standard case definitions, criteria for minimum data requirements, and emphasis on feedback through integrated forms, as well as research and training opportunities, are among the important tools available to improve the situation. Yet, efforts to establish fully more effective public health infrastructures may take a period of years to decades.

The aim in Africa is to identify a group of priority diseases categorized as epidemic-prone diseases, diseases targeted for eradication or elimination, and other diseases of public health importance. The challenge will be to integrate surveillance and epidemic preparedness and response activities for these priority diseases, especially when there are weakened ministries of health. Bilateral and multilateral agreements, as well as partnerships with nongovernmental organizations and commercial interests, are among the means being explored to strengthen disease surveillance and response activities, to transfer epidemiological and microbiological skills, and to facilitate timely recognition of these disease outbreaks and their control. Among the promising roles provided by global disease surveillance is the integration of new technology tools in resource-poor environments, such as in sub-Saharan Africa, for the development of an early-warning system based on remotely sensed (satellite) data for Rift Valley fever surveillance.

At a time when increasing attention is focused on many of the recently emerging infections (monkeypox virus, Rift Valley fever virus, *filiovirus, Vibrio cholerae* O139, and penicillin-resistant *Streptococcus pneumoniae*) and reemerging infectious diseases (malaria, tuberculosis, yellow fever, and trypanosomiasis) continually incubating and bursting forth from Africa, major gaps exist in surveillance, research and training programs, and the availability of qualified professionals concerned with infectious diseases in Africa. The infrastructure and level of support for surveillance, research, and training on emerging infectious diseases in Africa are extremely limited. There is a shrinking number of trained infectious disease specialists in Africa, from the community health worker, to the laboratory technician, to professionals in the specialized professions of virology, microbiology, medical entomology, epidemiology, and public health. The latter point was emphasized at the workshop on which this report is based, as none of the African scientists invited to make presentations at the workshop were available owing to exigent schedules and demanding workloads for the qualified few, in addition to difficulty in obtaining government permission to travel and technological obstacles to effective communication. The challenge ahead will be to broaden the base of qualified personnel at all levels in Africa.

INTEGRATED DISEASE SURVEILLANCE AND EPIDEMICS: PREPAREDNESS AND RESPONSE IN AFRICA

Bradley A. Perkins, M.D.
Chief, Meningitis and Special Pathogens Branch, National Center for Infectious Diseases, Centers for Disease Control and Prevention, United States

A project developed jointly by the World Health Organization (WHO), the African Regional Office of WHO, the Centers for Disease Control and Prevention (CDC), and the U.S. Agency for International Development (USAID) aims to improve the well-being of the approximately 600 million people currently residing in the 46 member states of the African Regional Office of WHO. The project implements integrated infectious disease surveillance and improved epidemic preparedness and response.

On September 2, 1998, the African Regional Office adopted a strategy for integrated epidemiological surveillance of diseases as a regional approach to control communicable diseases and urged its member states to evaluate surveillance and laboratory support, as well as to implement the regional strategy for integration as it was developed.

The response to smallpox has been used as a model for contemporary measures. Until the late 1960s, 10 to 15 million cases of smallpox occurred yearly and the overall smallpox mortality rate at a global level was 15 to 20 percent. Although the economic costs of the eradication effort were sizable, the benefits in terms of economics were similarly tremendous. Even for the smallpox initiative, which was relatively well funded, it took 2 years to establish effective surveillance in most areas.

The smallpox response model has been used, for example, to respond to meningitis in the sub-Saharan meningitis belt, where periodic, irregular, and large meningitis epidemics occur. A vaccine against meningitis is available, but it is ineffective in young children, so emergency mass campaigns are used to control the disease. Over the last decade, WHO, USAID, and other organizations have developed surveillance-based thresholds for the initiation of mass vaccinations, accompanied by appropriate laboratory confirmation. On the basis of some model data obtained over the last 10 years, it is known that a rapid response is essential for the effectiveness of this strategy.

Data from Ghana gathered in 1996 and 1997 suggest that about 5,000 cases of meningitis and 304 deaths were prevented by the reaction of the Ghana Ministry of Health. If 85 percent vaccine coverage could have been achieved within 1 week after the epidemic was identified, substantially more cases and deaths could have been avoided. These data provide an example of the effective use of surveillance data to detect a problem and also to assess the effectiveness of a public health response to that problem.

The difficulties with surveillance in Africa are well known. In the context of the multiple epidemics that have been recognized over the past decade, numerous assessments of surveillance systems have revealed problems essentially across the board.

Individuals who are part of vertically oriented programs at the national level and above try to communicate with district officials and health facilities at the local level, resulting in too much paperwork, too many different instructions, different terminologies, too many administrators, and conflicting priorities.

The time is right to move toward integrated disease surveillance and epidemic preparedness and response in Africa. A number of important things that leverage the opportunities for success in this area are happening. One of the first efforts was streamlining of the communication and conduct of public health surveillance, with the use of standard case definitions, minimum data requirements, and an emphasis on integrated forms, feedback, and training. No single approach is likely to fit all countries, yet WHO is committed to providing support to all of its member states.

The next major step was to identify a group of priority diseases. A group of 18 diseases was categorized. These included epidemic-prone diseases, diseases targeted for eradication or elimination, and other diseases of major public health importance. If effective surveillance is broken down into 10 elements, multiplied by 18 priority diseases, and combined with four levels of the health system, designing an ideal system becomes complex. All of these units require some technical input, and all must accommodate the other diseases included in the surveillance effort.

The transition to integration is happening. Most countries have existing systems for some disease surveillance. Recently, polio eradication has become a major focus of new efforts, which should establish an infrastructure for future responses. Surveillance for cholera, meningitis, neonatal tetanus, typhoid fever, yellow fever, dysentery, malaria, and measles is needed at various levels in many countries. Some countries, such as Tanzania, are requesting help with integrated disease surveillance. As development of public health infrastructures progresses over a period of years to decades, additional diseases can be added to the system. Currently, 15 polio laboratories are functioning, and 7 bacterial meningitis laboratories have been established, as have 5 diarrheal disease laboratories and 2 laboratories that are monitoring antimicrobial resistance.

Support from CDC for these efforts provides technical, epidemiological, and laboratory expertise in polio eradication and measles elimination programs, as well as in programs that address other vaccine-preventable childhood diseases; expansion of laboratory and technical capacity; development of training materials and other material support; and laboratory training and support. USAID and the United Nations Foundation have provided additional resources. National governments have exhibited a willingness to contribute actively to this effort.

The partners are in the process of defining indicators that would suggest progress and success. The level of integration of the current polio efforts are actively being measured. In addition, the number of outbreak investigations and the effectiveness of those responses are actively being monitored in a number of countries, and laboratory confirmation of suspected outbreaks is being obtained at the national level. The quality and frequency of feedback instruments are also being assessed. Clearly, improvements in communications technologies will aid these efforts. The key elements needed to design the ideal system and to develop the strategies for making the transition from existing systems to strengthened laboratory resources have been identified. Finally, the resources to begin this effort are available, but they are certainly not sufficient to sustain an effective system.

GLOBAL EMERGING INFECTIOUS DISEASES

Patrick W. Kelley, M.D., Dr. P.H.

Colonel and Director, Division of Preventive Medicine
Walter Reed Army Institute of Research, United States Army

A landmark 1992 Institute of Medicine report on emerging infections (IOM, 1992) resulted in the development of a CDC strategic plan for the nation, which suggested a specific role for the U. S. Department of Defense (DOD). Then, in 1996, President Bill Clinton issued a directive expanding the role of many federal agencies in global surveillance for infectious diseases, including DOD.

DOD's Expanded Role

DOD's role was expanded to include support of global surveillance, training, research, and response through centralized coordination. The DOD role includes improved preventive health programs for U.S. forces and their family members and enhanced involvement of military treatment facilities and laboratories in the United States and overseas. Beyond its health care infrastructure, DOD has some unique assets that it can bring to bear on the global problem of emerging infections.

A major asset is the DOD network of overseas laboratories in Egypt, Kenya, Thailand, Indonesia, and Peru. These are medical research and development laboratories that in some cases were established more than 50 years ago and that exist primarily for the purpose of product development. For example, the key studies conducted for the licensure of the hepatitis A and the Japanese encephalitis vaccines were done at these laboratories.

These laboratories have, in some instances, a biosafety level 3 capability. The laboratory in Cairo, Egypt, can if necessary, adapt to a biosafety level 4 capability. Although located in 5 countries, these laboratories have active research programs in about 31 countries; they have established extensive networks in their regions and have formal relationships with many ministries of health and the WHO.

The laboratories have tremendous depth. In almost every case they have expertise in virology, bacteriology, parasitology, other aspects of microbiology, veterinary medicine, and epidemiology. Although their primary purpose was to support product development, increasingly they are becoming involved with surveillance. In all, about 700 people work at these laboratories and are backed up by more than 800 more DOD scientists working on issues related to emerging infections.

The laboratories have additional assets: they are networked with state-of-the-art communications technologies and possess cutting-edge field diagnostic reagents that are field oriented, rapid, and invaluable in the response to emerging infectious diseases. In addition, the laboratories have access to special drugs and vaccines that might be of critical importance in regions with outbreaks of unusual pathogens.

Globally deployed military forces who are under medical surveillance are another unique asset. On any given day, U.S. troops are in the field in more than 70 countries. Because they are under intense medical surveillance, they provide a key opportunity to document the emergence of new conditions. The DOD serum repository is a valuable source of sera from subjects before and after disease development. These sera can be used to document exposures to various infectious agents. Currently, DOD has more than 25 million catalogued specimens from DOD personnel.

A major focus at DOD overseas laboratories is drug-resistant malaria. This is because DOD operates the largest malaria drug development program in the world and needs up-to-date information on resistance patterns. DOD also has a surveillance program for antibiotic-resistant enteric agents and for hemorrhagic fevers, including dengue, and influenza. In addition, DOD supports regional syndromic sentinel surveillance networks.

Currently, DOD is trying to support WHO's efforts to link military public health laboratories together to conduct surveillance on antibiotic resistance or other types of medical surveillance. Military hospitals often serve as a good source of surveillance data in less developed countries because of the quality of their facilities.

DOD Involvement in Rift Valley Fever Outbreak

An example of recent DOD involvement in Africa was the outbreak of Rift Valley fever in 1997–1998 in East Africa. Approximately 80,000 people ultimately contracted Rift Valley fever, resulting in hundreds of deaths. In addition to the direct toll on the human population, there was a tremendous toll on the animal population in this pastoral economy. Using its laboratory in Kenya, DOD was able to quickly assist with the initial epidemiological and entomological investigations. At the time that the outbreak surfaced Kenya had no laboratory capacity for the diagnosis of Rift Valley fever. Specimens had to be sent to either South Africa or CDC to make the diagnosis. Using resources at its laboratory in Cairo, DOD was able to quickly transfer technology for rapid diagnosis to Kenya so that the outbreak could be defined rapidly and locally. Experts in remote sensing also collected data to establish indicators that are evident at least 3 or 4 months before outbreaks. In the future this will enable the government to initiate immunizations for animals and thus prevent the amplification of the virus and its transmission to humans. DOD also provided access to the Rift Valley fever vaccine for at-risk laboratory workers in Kenya.

Syndromic Surveillance in Indonesia

DOD is also establishing a syndromic surveillance system, called the Early Warning Outbreak Recognition System (EWORS), in Indonesia. Several sites around the Indonesian archipelago once every 24 hours report syndromic data to a central point in Jakarta, where a DOD laboratory is collocated with the Indonesian Ministry of Health. The system is focused on hospitals located around Indonesia, where nurses collect syndromic data from patients. These data are entered into a database where one can enter not only the signs and symptoms but also the specific working diagnosis. In almost real time the frequencies of various syndromes can be tracked across the archipelago.

Integrating Surveillance in the Caribbean

A different approach to infectious disease surveillance is under way in the Caribbean, in collaboration with PAHO's Caribbean Epidemiology Center (CAREC). In 1997, CAREC brought together the national epidemiologists and laboratory directors from its 21 member countries and said that by the year 2000 they wanted to have in place a surveillance system capable of monitoring trends and impacts of emerging infectious diseases and providing timely, relevant, and accurate feedback. The concept was one of hierarchical, laboratory-based surveillance, with CAREC the regional pinnacle of the hierarchy.

DOD donated equipment for a website to CAREC so that it can receive data from its member countries and report back to them. DOD then sponsored a meeting of the 21 countries for a week of training in the use of automated equipment and other aspects of informatics for public health reporting. Each independent country took home two computers. Subsequently, DOD is providing additional equipment to each independent country and an additional week of training to further support the surveillance system. The reporting system is based on CDC's Public Health Laboratory Information System (PHLIS). The PHLIS program is capable of integrating into one system reports from multiple types of reporting.

Facilitating Training and Capacity Building

DOD laboratories also serve as training sites, offering a number of courses in outbreak investigation, for example, throughout Southeast Asia. The aim is to transfer epidemiological and microbiological skills and to facilitate timely recognition of outbreaks and control. These courses should also bring some uniformity to the outbreak investigation process.

In countries with weaker ministries of health, such as some African nations, DOD has increasingly turned to nongovernmental organizations and commercial organizations, such as the African Medical and Research Foundation and the African Conservation Company, to establish partnerships.

EMERGING INFECTIONS IN AFRICA:
THE WHO RESPONSE

Guénaël Rodier, M.D.
Department of Communicable Disease Surveillance and Response
World Health Organization, Geneva

There is a dire need for global surveillance of emerging infectious diseases, including in the African region. Strengthening of national surveillance systems is an important part of improving global surveillance. From this perspective the World Health Organization (WHO) assists countries with the development of national surveillance plans and surveillance standards on the basis of selected priority diseases and by use of an integrated or multidisease approach. WHO also supports epidemiology training in the field to ensure a better capacity for preparedness and response to epidemics at the national and regional levels. In addition, WHO continues to strengthen global laboratory surveillance networks, including the antimicrobial resistance network and the hemorrhagic fever surveillance network. Military networks and the Pasteur Institutes network are examples of non-disease-specific global networks, also important partners of WHO. The revision of the International Health Regulations is another important element of the WHO strategy in global surveillance and control of emerging infections.

On the response side, WHO supports a rapid epidemic response team and other global response networks such as the International Coordinating Group, which ensures that vaccines and other resources are delivered in an equitable manner during meningococcal meningitis epidemics, and the WHO Cholera Task Force, which focuses on cholera and other epidemic diarrheal diseases.

Global Epidemic Intelligence

In the area of epidemiological surveillance of emerging infections, there have been a number of new approaches, such as integrated (or multidisease) surveillance, syndromic reporting, and the development of Internet-based disease surveillance.

Global Epidemic Intelligence, established at WHO in 1996, was created to improve international preparedness and the international response to epidemics by sharing the same information in a timely fashion. It also plays an essential role in countering confusing information that can have a major impact on international travel and trade. Through active collection of information on ongoing or rumored outbreaks worldwide and rapid verification of theses reports, WHO is able to provide valuable and timely information to the international public health community.

This system requires multiple skills, not only in epidemiology, infectious diseases, and laboratory surveillance but also skills in international public health and field experience, telecommunications and informatics, and information management. It also requires partnership with the public and private sectors. Six regional offices of WHO, such as the African Regional Office (AFRO), play an essential role in this network, particularly for verification purposes, as they have privileged access to countries.

Use of the Internet

The Internet is an increasing source of outbreak-related information. For example, information can be obtained through news on media wires, electronic discussion groups, and various websites. Epidemic intelligence must take in to account the unrestricted use of the new technologies, such as the Internet and the increased participation in the health fields by nongovernmental organizations and private-sector interests, whose activities and information often bypass official reporting systems. This is a new situation and can allow additional time for proper action to be taken in advance to avert panic and minimize potential damage to trade.

To explore the extent to which nontraditional means of reporting, particularly over the Internet, can be channeled to good use, WHO developed with the Canadian Ministry of Health a computer application (Global Public Health Intelligence Network) that scans hundreds of websites and media wires 10 times a day for information that could be associated with reports of communicable diseases or disasters. Of the 450 reports of outbreaks verified in the past 2.5 years, more than 50 percent have come from the media.

Disease Distribution and Verification

The reports gathered from websites are verified and entered into a database that also contains data from other reporting sources. The information is then mapped, sometimes down to the village level (WHO/United Nations Children's Fund HealthMap Programme).

Retrospective analysis of the data shows that diarrheal diseases—in particular, cholera—are the most frequently reported events. For the last 3 years cholera has been the most frequently reported event in the African region. Meningococcal meningitis, acute hemorrhagic fever syndromes, acute neurological syndromes, acute respiratory syndromes, yellow fever, and plague are also frequently reported. About 60 percent of all the reports processed by the WHO outbreak verification group come from the so-called emergency countries, that is, countries experiencing civil strife, civil war, and economic collapse.

The first step in the verification process is to share the report with the ministry of health of the relevant country so that it may investigate and initiate a possible response. Nongovernmental organizations and the United Nations network are important partners in outbreak verification. When an event is sufficiently verified and if it is likely to have international implications (likely spread to other countries, impact on international travel and trade, or requests for international assistance), it is shared through the weekly Outbreak Verification List (OVL) with WHO partners in international public health. The OVL reports the presented syndrome or disease, the location of the event, its source, the available figures and number of reported cases and deaths, and the contact details for WHO professionals who are monitoring this particular event. When an event is fully verified and when there is a need for public information, it is described on the WHO website and other websites and its description is published in the *Weekly Epidemiological Record*.

Verification can be difficult because of limited infrastructure and human resources in a country, poor communications systems, a lack of laboratory capacity, and civil conflict and war situations, which are increasingly common.

Outbreak Response Role of WHO

WHO responds to epidemics at the request of its member states. After WHO receives a request, its role is to mobilize the international response and to coordinate the response when there are different partners from different regions. Coordination is necessary for field activities, logistics, information vis-à-vis the media, contact with national authorities, and the raising of emergency funds. The response can be limited by a delay in the initial request, insufficient preparedness, time pressures, bilateral agreements that could impede coordination, and concerns for security in the field. In addition, the partners, either nongovernmental organizations or major laboratories, sometimes compete over visibility and access to clinical specimens and scientific data. When an outbreak is over, WHO should then ensure that there is a national follow-up plan, particularly in the area of epidemic preparedness and surveillance. Specific guidelines on how to handle certain types of outbreaks have also been developed, including videos, particularly targeting epidemic diseases specific to Africa, such as Ebola hemorrhagic fever.

4

Emerging Infections in Asia and the Pacific Region

OVERVIEW

The trend toward globalization of the economy is most evident across Asia, Australia, and the Pacific region. Common political interests are among the driving forces bringing together countries in Asia, along with the United States, and other countries in the Pacific region. However, obstacles to globalization exist in the region. Among these are public health problems, which are often at the heart of the political and economic challenges to globalization. For example, a number of important global diseases, such as influenza, dengue, Japanese encephalitis, tuberculosis, and pneumonia, are endemic to the region, as are the newly emerging Hendra and Nipah viruses.

Although the emerging infectious disease problems facing countries in the Asia-Pacific region are as great as those facing countries elsewhere, the potential for the prevention and mitigation of disease outbreaks in the region is noteworthy, as evidenced by several recent epidemic threats. The region is fortunate to have access to advances in electronic communications, infectious disease epidemiology, and laboratory techniques, together with resources for training and for maintenance and enhancement of the public health infrastructure.

EMERGING INFECTIOUS DISEASES IN HONG KONG
AND THEIR PUBLIC HEALTH SIGNIFICANCE

Kwok Hang Mak, M.B., M.Sc.
Consultant, Community Medicine, Department of Health
Hong Kong Special Administrative Region, People's Republic of China

In recent years, the Hong Kong Special Administrative Region of the People's Republic of China has witnessed, like other parts of the world, the emergence and reemergence of various infectious diseases, in particular influenza, cholera, and enterovirus infections. This region is particularly vulnerable to infectious diseases because it is densely populated (6.68 million people in 1998), is in the crossroads between the East and the West, encounters a heavy volume of international travel, and has live poultry markets in close proximity to residential areas.

Influenza A Virus (H5N1)

In 1997, a total of 18 cases of human infection with influenza A virus subtype H5N1, which was previously known to infect birds only, occurred in Hong Kong. The first case appeared in May 1997; the remaining cases occurred in November and December 1997. They involved 8 males and 10 females ages 1 to 60 years. Half of the cases occurred among children at or under age 12. All of the patients presented with a high temperature and a sore throat; the majority also developed a cough. Six individuals died as a result of viral pneumonia and multiorgan failure. Genetic sequencing confirmed the avian origins of the viruses isolated from patients. Results of an investigation indicated that the main mode of transmission was from bird to human. Human-to-human transmission was documented but was found to be relatively inefficient and uncommon. Epidemiological studies showed that the major risk factor was visiting poultry stalls in a market the week before the onset of illness.

In view of the evidence that the H5N1 virus affected chickens in the local community, a slaughtering exercise was launched on December 29, 1997; a total of 1.5 million poultry were killed. This measure effectively brought the outbreak to an end. A whole host of measures was introduced to ensure that the poultry sold in local markets were safe. They included quarantine and testing of imported chickens, segregation of chickens from ducks and geese, and improvement of hygienic conditions in the markets. Close attention to surveillance of humans and animals for evidence of influenza was maintained while preparation of pandemic plans and the development of vaccine and antiviral agents continued.

This outbreak illustrates the importance of a robust public health infrastructure for disease surveillance and the need for international efforts and multidisciplinary collaboration to address the threat of influenza. Apart from disease prevention and control, due consideration should also be given to the economic and political impacts of such an outbreak, as well as to the communication strategies used during a disease outbreak.

Avian H9N2 Viruses

In April 1999, avian subtype H9N2 viruses were isolated from two young girls ages 1 and 4, but only the older girl had a history of exposure to chickens. Both girls recovered completely from influenza-like illnesses. Investigation results also suggested that the main mode of transmission was from bird to human, although the possibility of human-to-human transmission remained open. In view of the low prevalence of antibodies among various study groups, the satisfactory outcomes of the cases, and the fact that the virus—although commonly found in poultry—usually caused mild symptoms, there was ample evidence to conclude that the discovery of this H9N2 virus in humans did not appear to pose an imminent threat to public health.

Swine Influenza A Virus (H3N2)

Another discovery new to Hong Kong in the arena of influenza occurred in October 1999. An influenza A virus subtype H3N2 isolated from a 10-month-old girl was proved by overseas reference laboratories to have originated in swine. The patient had a mild influenza-like illness and made a full recovery. Investigations did not reveal any history of exposure to pigs or poultry by the patient or her family members. Initial blood tests also showed that the family members were not exposed to this swine flu virus. Although this reflects the sensitivity of the local influenza surveillance system, it further reinforces the importance of veterinary surveillance in animals, including pigs and birds.

Conclusion

The discovery of avian and swine influenza virus infections among humans in Hong Kong has driven home a strong message that vigilance in public health surveillance of human and animal populations is indispensable. Many emerging infectious diseases, like influenza, are zoonotic problems, and their control requires a close and effective collaboration between public health and veterinary workers. As surveillance increases, it is likely that more avian influenza virus isolates will be identified, linking research issues to public policy. It is the concerted efforts of individuals across different disciplines and boundaries that provide the winning edge.

EMERGING DISEASES IN THE AUSTRALASIAN REGION

John S. Mackenzie, Ph.D.
Professor and Head, Department of Microbiology and Parasitology,
The University of Queensland, Brisbane, Australia

Emerging diseases in Australia are, with a few important exceptions, not dissimilar in their identity, occurrence, and patterns of incidence to those described in developed countries elsewhere. Most of the exceptions are either vector-borne or zoonotic viral diseases, and they fall into two patterns: known diseases that are increasing in incidence or geographical spread and novel diseases that had not previously been recognized. The former include mosquito-borne virus diseases, such as disease caused by Japanese encephalitis (JE) virus, dengue viruses, and Barmah Forest virus, whereas the latter are zoonotic diseases, such as those caused by Hendra virus, Menangle virus, and Australian bat lyssavirus (ABL).

Japanese Encephalitis Virus

Of the mosquito-borne viral diseases, the greatest threat to Australia and nearby Pacific islands is undoubtedly that caused by JE virus. To date there have been five clinical cases of JE: four on Badu Island in the Torres Strait and one in Cape York on the Australian mainland. The first three cases occurred on Badu Island in 1995, whereas the fourth case occurred on Badu Island and the fifth case occurred on the Australian mainland in 1998. There have been almost 60 virus isolations from mosquitoes and pigs. All but one of the mosquito isolates was from *Culex annulirostris* mosquitoes. The first outbreak, in 1995, was driven by the close proximity to human habitation of mosquitoes and their breeding habitats and by the widespread practice of keeping pigs in backyards. The second outbreak, in 1998, was believed to have been associated with an extensive drought in Papua New Guinea (PNG), which led to increased mosquito breeding as rivers began to dry into stagnant pools. Australia has suitable vertebrate hosts (feral pigs and ardeid birds) and vectors (*Cx. annulirostris*) by which JE becomes enzootic. Of some concern is that fruit bats might be potential vertebrate hosts in both rural and urban settings.

The virus is now widespread in PNG and is threatening to move farther east, toward the Solomon Islands. The first four clinical cases of JE in PNG were recognized in 1997 and 1998, and two mosquito isolates were obtained. Molecular epidemiological studies showed that the Australian and PNG virus isolates were almost identical, indicating that the source of the Australian outbreaks was PNG.

After the 1995 outbreak, the JE vaccine (Biken) was offered to inhabitants of the central and northern islands of the Torres Strait. Approximately 9,000 doses of vaccine were distributed. In addition, sentinel pigs were established on several islands in the Torres Strait and on the Australian mainland near Bamega. There was widespread seroconversion in these pigs during the 1998 outbreak. Surveillance of humans and pigs has continued to the present. The spread of JE to the Australian zoogeographic region may have occurred by a number of means, including natural spread through eastern Indonesia by means of mosquito-pig or mosquito-bird transmission cycles, human travel and transmigration, and airlifts of pigs to indigenous people.

Dengue

All four types of dengue virus have been introduced into the dengue-receptive areas of northeastern Australia over the past decade, and epidemics caused by three serotypes of dengue virus have occurred. Humans are the only vertebrate hosts; when an epidemic subsides, the virus disappears and must be reintroduced, probably via viremic travelers returning to Australia or through the movement of people across the Torres Strait. The only vector in Australia is *Aedes aegypti*, whose range extends over most of northern Queensland, Australia.

The management plan for control includes rapid reporting of cases and subsequent vector control. In a 4-year period (1995 to 1998), 31 reports of dengue came from general practitioners, public hospitals doctors, private laboratories, or Queensland Health Scientific Services. It was determined that the countries of origin included PNG, Indonesia, Thailand, the Philippines, and Vietnam.

Other Emerging Diseases

Barmah Forest virus is an alphavirus only found in Australia. It has been recognized as a human pathogen for about 13 years, but it has recently been shown to have spread into new areas of Australia. Its vertebrate hosts are believed to be marsupials, especially small species. It was first isolated from mosquitoes captured in southeast Australia in 1974. The Barmah Forest virus causes a disease syndrome similar to that caused by another Australian alphavirus, the Ross River virus, which is found throughout Australia. The Ross River virus has been referred to such a virus in some reports, but it does not fully fall into the definition of as an emerging virus. Although the incidence of Ross River virus infection has indeed increased slightly in recent years, this may largely be due to population increases and changes in demography.

Of the novel zoonotic diseases, Hendra virus was the first to be recognized during an outbreak in race horses in Brisbane in 1994. This was shown to be a natural virus of fruit bats, and to be widely distributed in northern and eastern Australia, as well as PNG. Hendra virus has been classified as the first member of a new genus in the family *Paramyxoviridae*. Studies of Hendra virus led to the discovery of ABL, a rabies virus-like virus, in both fruit bats and at least one species of insectivorous bat. ABL belongs to antigenic group 1 of the lyssaviruses, which is the same group to which classical rabies virus belongs, but ABL and rabies virus can be differentiated on genetic grounds. The virus most recently detected in Australia, Menangle virus, was recognized as the cause of an increased incidence of fetal death in a commercial piggery and as a possible cause of an influenza-like illness in humans. It also appears to be a virus of fruit bats and is a member of the *Rubalavirus* genus in the family *Paramyxoviridae*.

The discovery of three new zoonotic viruses from fruit bats in Australia is of wider interest, as fruit bat populations overlap from the Pacific islands through Australia, southern Asia, and possibly into the Middle East and Africa. Thus, for any virus found in Australia, related viruses will probably exist throughout the range of similar bats. The first of these may be Nipah virus, which was recently discovered in Malaysia.

There have been other examples of emerging diseases in Australia, such as the occurrence of waterborne epidemics due to *Cryptosporidium parvum* in eastern Australia, and an increased incidence of enterohemorrhagic *Escherichia coli* belonging to serotype O111:H, which is associated with hemolytic-uremic syndrome. Australia has also had a recent emerging problem with community-acquired strains of methicillin-resistant *Staphylococcus aureus* (cMRSA). These strains of MRSA appear to have arisen in two distinct areas. One strain appears to have initially developed and spread in northern, western, and southern Australia, whereas a strain known to be a Western Samoan strain, which appears to have developed in the South Pacific, then became a problem in New Zealand and is now found in eastern Australia. The significance is that the standard antibiotics that are given for therapy (e.g., flucloxacillin) are ineffective and it takes 48 hours for a laboratory to confirm that the isolate is resistant. Hence, patients with serious infections may be receiving ineffective antibiotics for 48 hours. MRSA is still relatively infrequent (less than 1 percent of *S. aureus* isolates in eastern Australia). However in certain areas of Auckland, New Zealand, more than 10 percent of community-acquired *S. aureus* infections are now caused by cMRSA.

The importance of epizootics in wildlife is of growing concern because of their possible zoonotic potential. Indeed, in recent years most novel emerging diseases have been zoonotic diseases. Thus, there is a recognition of the necessity for improved infectious disease surveillance in humans. However, there is also a need to undertake surveillance of infectious diseases in wild and domestic animals and a need for public education and awareness of the possibility of transmission of diseases from wildlife to humans. Finally, the experiences gained with emerging infectious diseases in Australia have clearly indicated that disease surveillance should be undertaken as a regional, multinational activity.

INTERNATIONAL SMART PARTNERSHIP IN EMERGING DISEASES: SENSE AND SENSITIVITY

Sai-Kit Lam, M.Sc., Ph.D.

Professor and Head, Department of Medical Microbiology, Faculty of Medicine, University of Malaya, Kuala Lumpur, Malaysia

Introduction

The World Health Organization (WHO) estimates that infectious diseases account for more than 17 million deaths per year worldwide and that at least 30 new infectious diseases have emerged within the last two decades. The world's 6 billion people are at risk for many endemic diseases, with the most populated and economically depressed countries in Southeast Asia at highest risk (Lam, 1998). There are inadequate funds, personnel, resources, and political commitment in developing countries to adopt the WHO Resolution of 1995, urging member countries to commit to an international program for the worldwide monitoring and control of infectious diseases.

Emerging infections can arise in countries in Asia and the Pacific. The emergence of the avian influenza A virus serves as an example of the need for strengthened surveillance of emerging diseases in this part of the world. Other viruses that should be placed on the "watch list" include yellow fever—because of the presence of its vector in the region—and the African hemorrhagic fevers, because of increased trade and traffic among countries of these regions.

Many viruses responsible for emerging infections already may exist in Southeast Asian countries, but because of the lack of surveillance and diagnostic capabilities, their existence may have gone unnoticed. Hantaviruses in Malaysia provide an example: Since the 1980s, there have been only three publications providing evidence of the existence of hantavirus in humans and rodents. Interest in hantaviruses recently was revived when, with the help of South Korea, we obtained serological evidence of hantavirus infections in 4 of 119 patients with chronic renal failure. Additional serological evidence in rodents indicated that there might be more than one member of the hantavirus family lurking in Malaysia. Virus isolation from lungs and other tissues of seropositive rodents is underway.

Emerging infections pose a serious problem in Malaysia, as evidenced by three outbreaks of unknown viral etiology in the relatively short period of two years. International assistance was sought and the help rendered was greatly appreciated. Many lessons were learned in the handling of these outbreaks and the unexpected problems that occurred. It is hoped that by sharing our experiences, we can obtain a greater understanding of investigations and, with hope, establish a better international "smart partnership" in future.

Emerging Infections in Malaysia

The first outbreak took place in 1997 in Sarawak, East Malaysia, and subsequently spread to peninsular Malaysia. The outbreak in Sarawak was investigated by local scientists and by the U.S. Centers for Disease Control and Prevention (CDC). Thirty-four children between the ages of 5 months and 7 years died with cardiac and central nervous system involvement. The early diagnosis announced by the Ministry of Health was Coxsackie B myocarditis. When similar cases were seen and investigated in Peninsular Malaysia, enterovirus 71 (EV71) was isolated from the brain stem in 4 fatal cases (Lam et al., 1998). This finding was supported by immunohistochemical staining (Wong et al., 1999). Outbreaks of EV71 in Taiwan (Huang et al., 1999) and Australia subsequently provided further evidence of the neurovirulence of this enterovirus strain. However, a recent paper from Sarawak disputed the finding of EV71 as the cause of the Malaysian outbreak, claiming that the deaths were due to viral myocarditis and caused by subgenus B adenovirus (Cardosa et al., 1999).

The second outbreak took place in early 1999. Over 100 cases of fever, arthralgia, and arthritis were reported by the local press in a squatter settlement where sanitation was poor and there was an abundance of *Aedes aegypti.* Dengue and other known viral infections were excluded. With the help of Australia, the cause of the outbreak was found to be due to chikungunya virus, a virus hitherto unknown locally, but prevalent in neighboring countries. It is speculated that the virus was introduced into the country through migrant workers. Since Malaysia is heavily dependent on a migrant workforce, it is anticipated that other emerging infections will be introduced into the country.

The third outbreak also was of viral encephalitis and thought to be Japanese encephalitis (JE), an endemic, seasonal disease. For five months it was treated as a JE outbreak and control measures included vector control and vaccination against JE Despite these efforts the disease spread to several states in Malaysia as well as to Singapore. Of the 265 clinical cases reported among pig farm workers, 105 died and there were neurological sequelae and relapses in a few who recovered. A new paramyxovirus related to the Australian Hendra virus was isolated, and with the help of CDC it was confirmed to be a new virus (Chua et al., 1999). It was named Nipah virus after the village from which the patient came. Because of the earlier misdiagnosis of JE, the whole issue was politicized and played up by the press and public media, creating a difficult situation for the investigators.

Lessons Learned

In developing countries, there are seldom enough funds, personnel, or resources to conduct outbreak investigation. Thus, there is reliance on international agencies for assistance. Such assistance, which is usually on a government-to-government basis, is much appreciated. In the Nipah outbreak international assistance came from many countries, including the United States, Australia, Japan, Taiwan, and Germany. However, unexpected problems can arise due to failure to recognize and appreciate cultural, religious, and political sensitivities.

Because of the tragic loss of lives and livelihoods during the Nipah outbreak, there was considerable pressure brought to bear by political parties on both local and international experts. It is imperative that investigators not get caught in the quagmire of intrigue and become political pawns.

One area that was poorly handled was publicity. The Nipah outbreak created international interest, some unfortunately sensationalistic. There were also some biased comments and reporting by critics not involved in the investigation. Foreign press releases caused embarrassment to the local government because of contradicting data and viewpoints. It is important to release accurate information during the outbreak, preferably from a single source. Misleading statements can lead to confusion, anguish, and fear in an already tense situation.

The electronic media have an important role to play in the fight against emerging infections. During the EV71 and Nipah outbreaks, offers of help came in quickly, a true advantage. However, rapid communication also can be abused, as was all too evident in the Nipah outbreak when the issue was politicized and used to cast aspersions on those handling the outbreak.

After the Nipah outbreak an international meeting was held to discuss areas of future research. There was some pressure to include Nipah virus as a strict P4 agent, which effectively would prevent any further work with the virus in Malaysia. This was a sensitive issue, but fortunately good sense prevailed and a compromise was reached. The final recommendation was to allow this highly pathogenic virus to be handled at the highest level of biosafety possible, with responsible national authorities developing appropriate policies and guidelines for laboratory procedures.

Two years after the Sarawak outbreak there remains a difference of opinion about the cause of death and the etiologic agent responsible. The findings have yet to be released by those called in to assist in the investigation, thus prolonging the confusion.

Rapid response is an important component in the fight against emerging infections. Many countries are ill prepared for rapid response. Recent events in Malaysia have highlighted the need to strengthen this aspect of public health. The Ministry of Health has formed a permanent committee to identify weaknesses in the system and proposals for change. In addition, a new Infectious Disease Center has been established and will be equipped with adequate facilities to handle future emerging diseases outbreaks.

Transfer of appropriate technology to developing countries from foreign experts is most important. In the Nipah outbreak, CDC and the Australian Animal Health Laboratory were instrumental in helping set up diagnostic capabilities and generously provided the necessary reagents.

Following the outbreak, there is usually much interest in continued research and data analyses on the materials gathered. Research priorities should be developed by giving equal consideration to all of the international partners to avoid dissension over proprietary rights to clinical materials and authorship of publications. "Smart partnership" requires total trust and transparency in all aspects of the investigation; there should be no hidden agendas. Open communication should be established and misunderstandings ironed out to prevent frustration and unwarranted accusation.

In summary, emerging infection is something we have to live with for years to come. Developing countries usually serve as the epicenter, and yet they are not equipped to handle outbreak investigation without international assistance. Such investigations must be conducted in a "smart partnership" agreement to promote cooperation to achieve public health.

5

Emerging Infections in Europe

OVERVIEW

The realization of the "global village" is most evident in Europe, as barriers to travel, commerce, and information sharing among countries are removed. However, Europe is not one country, and many of the states that comprised the former Soviet Union are actually located in central Asia. A challenge for Europe lies in how best to integrate local needs with national, political, and international needs when it comes to disease surveillance and response. The need for a clearer understanding of local requirements and the need for leadership behind the issues, followed by critical assessment and strategic planning for infrastructure development for infectious disease surveillance and response systems, are as evident in Europe as elsewhere. Yet, legal barriers or legal implications for building or implementation of such disease surveillance systems abound. Some countries may believe that these efforts could undermine their ability to protect the health of their citizenry or to retain state sovereignty. Some countries may be concerned about the diminishment of state authority within their own territories. International and national laws must be understood and discussed in the context of establishing cooperative efforts and meeting local needs for strategic planning in terms of infectious diseases. The Europe-wide EntreNet is one example of cooperation and coordination across political and geographical boundaries for the prevention and control of human salmonellosis and other food-borne illnesses in Europe.

PANDEMIC STRATEGIC PLANNING

Jane Leese, M.D.
Senior Medical Officer, Immunization Team
Department of Health, London

The Institute of Medicine (1992) defined emerging and reemerging infectious diseases as those "diseases of infectious origin whose incidence in humans has increased within the past two decades, or threatens to increase in the near future." This definition is wide, encompassing not only new entities, but also new incidents or outbreaks of established diseases with public health implications, changing trends, and diseases that have increased in importance because of, for example, the actual or potential emergence of antimicrobial resistance.

Diseases appear on the national or international political agenda for a variety of reasons: (1) new scientific evaluations clearly demonstrate a risk or potential risk to public health (this may not, however, be enough on its own); (2) a sudden, rather than an insidious, onset of an infectious disease; (3) preconceived perceptions of a disease (e.g., the outbreak of plague in India in 1994 was associated with international hysteria out of proportion to the risk on the basis of preconceived notions of the Black Death and other historical incidents); (4) a risk to trade or tourism; (5) extensive media coverage; (6) powerful lobbies at work; or (7) the issuance of an authoritative report from a respected body. A variety of reasons then affect how long a disease stays on the agenda, many of which are not necessarily scientifically or clinically appropriate. Another influence is cost. For example, in the United Kingdom a report from the National Audit Office on the cost to the National Health Service of hospital-acquired infections is likely to focus action on such infections as a developing priority.

Pandemic Influenza Contingency Plan in the United Kingdom

The study of influenza has provided useful experience in planning for an emerging infectious disease. In the United Kingdom it has been estimated that some 3,000 to 4,000 people die from influenza every year. In 1989, the most severe of recent epidemics, it was estimated that 26,000 people died from an influenza-related illness during the 6 to 8 weeks of the epidemic. Drawing on the experience and on experiences with previous pandemics of the last century, the United Kingdom has developed a national pandemic influenza contingency plan. The plan defines the roles and responsibilities of all the organizations and people who would be involved in the response to a new pandemic. What first emerges from this exercise is the large number of people who would be involved in the response and therefore the need for strong coordination.

The plan moves in phases, from the interpandemic period, through recognition of a new strain with pandemic potential, to outbreaks of illness outside the United Kingdom, outbreaks within the United Kingdom, the pandemic stage itself, and then the end of the pandemic, when the whole response would be reviewed. The World Health Organization (WHO) has since published guidance on planning for a pandemic. Currently, the effort is to bring the plan for the United Kingdom into concordance with the WHO plan.

There are five important and parallel strategies within the plan for the United Kingdom. The first concerns surveillance so that the country is in the best position to identify new strains of influenza and monitor their geographic spread. The second concerns vaccine development and supply and the development and implementation of vaccination policies. The third strategy concerns communications plans. The fourth concerns managing the burden of disease when it arises and the accompanying disruption to health and other services, and the fifth component is research.

The Hong Kong Influenza A Virus Outbreak

The outbreak of avian influenza A virus subtype H5N1 in Hong Kong in 1997 put the plan for the United Kingdom to its most recent test. The speed at which the outbreak became widely publicly reported led to some initial confusion about its nature and the size of the geographical area through which it was spreading, emphasizing the importance of a strong communications strategy. The United Kingdom was fortunate in that the WHO laboratory based in London was able to provide authoritative information during these early stages. Critical also was the high level of organization in Hong Kong, including the timely establishment of a website, updated at a specified time daily. Within the United Kingdom another early issue was whether surveillance was sufficient to detect cases in the United Kingdom should they be imported. General practitioners in areas of the country with large Chinese populations were asked to be alert to new cases of influenza-like illness and to send samples for investigation.

Another early part of the response was establishment of laboratory facilities suitable for work on the virus and the development of reagents. One problem not anticipated in the plan for the United Kingdom was that the Hong Kong virus was of avian origin. Thus, the Ministry of Agriculture needed to be involved and was rightly concerned about both the importation of the virus and proper containment in the laboratories handling it. The laboratories had to increase their containment facilities. Occupational health policy was a further consideration: should staff working on the virus take amantadine prophylactically? Another early issue to be considered was whether assistance should be sent to Hong Kong. This extended to how Europe might in the future better support WHO in its response to international outbreaks.

One lesson from this incident was that vaccine production during a pandemic may present unforeseen complexities and take longer than planned. On this occasion, the virus was so virulent that it killed the ferrets in which it was inoculated as well as the eggs in which it was to grow. One possible vaccine strain was identified, but it was still highly virulent and could not be grown under usual manufacturing conditions. A government-funded laboratory with suitable containment facilities was employed to produce a batch of virus to make sufficient vaccine for early clinical trials. This would have presented problems had manufacture on a large scale been required.

European Response to Emerging Infectious Diseases

Within Europe, considerable progress has been made in recent years to improve preparedness and the response to emerging infectious diseases. In September 1998, the European Parliament and Council passed a decision to set up a network for the epidemiological surveillance and control of communicable diseases in the community. This effort, which became active in July 1999, required the linking of national surveillance centers as well as administrations responsible for public health. The system builds on an established set of networks for surveillance of individual diseases, such as travel-related Legionnaires' disease, EntreNet (for enteric organisms), human immunodeficiency virus infection (HIV)/AIDS, tuberculosis, and drug resistance. Additional work has been undertaken to underpin the network. National surveillance institutes have collaborated in looking at standards and priorities for surveillance. A highly successful field epidemiology training program, called the European Programme for Intervention Epidemiology Training (EPIET), has been established. This has not only provided a cadre of people with expertise in handling international incidents, but has also facilitated international collaborations through regular contacts among EPIET instructors and trainees.

Regular surveillance bulletins in both paper and electronic form, have been produced. In addition, inventories of the available capacities and capabilities across Europe have been generated.

One important component of this new network is that it puts the public health authorities, usually the ministries of health, in communication with each other. The first priority for this part of the network has been to set up an early-warning system, whereby secure messages are shared as soon as a potential problem arises. In the long term, greater discussion over appropriate control measures will also be required of the network, although these measures remain the responsibility of individual member states.

Importance of Local Surveillance and Collaboration

Although cross-national cooperation is important, its success depends on the quality of local surveillance. In early-warning and response systems, the local level is required to serve a disease intelligence function and needs the ability to assess possible indicator events (e.g., changes in over-the-counter drug sales at pharmacies, school absenteeism, as well as the data generated from more conventional disease surveillance activities). Many emerging infections are zoonotic in origin. Surveillance systems at the local level must thus work closely with agricultural and veterinary colleagues and those undertaking surveillance in other related fields. Surveillance systems must be flexible to adapt, for example, to changing patterns of health care. The trend, for example, towards the use of near-patient diagnosis or the use of advice lines instead of a visit to a general practitioner's office could result in the loss of valuable surveillance data unless the new systems are adapted to the activities required for infectious disease surveillance. All surveillance increasingly needs to be undertaken with due attention to protection of patient confidentiality and privacy. If preparedness for emerging infectious diseases is to be maintained, surveillance systems need to be reviewed and adapted at regular intervals at the local, national, and international levels.

A VIEW FROM THE GROUND: TUBERCULOSIS AS AN EXAMPLE OF A REEMERGING INFECTIOUS DISEASE IN THE FORMER SOVIET UNION

Ian Small, M.A.
Head of Mission, Médecins sans Frontières
Tashkent, Uzbekistan

Introduction

In the aftermath of the Cold War, a diverse group of 15 independent countries—with a population of more than 350 million people, dozens of different languages, and just as many different ethnic and national groups—faced the reemergence of the tuberculosis (TB) bacillus. TB stands above all emerging infections as the single largest public health concern in the region. Various factors affect the response to this threat, including economic, environmental, and political elements, the infrastructure and the capacity of the stricken communities to respond, diagnostic and treatment considerations and constraints, and the role of nongovernmental organizations (NGOs) in combating TB.

This summary focuses on the situation in five Central Asian states that were part of the former Soviet Union (FSU)—Kazakhstan, Uzbekistan, Kyrgyzstan, Turkmenistan, and Tajikistan—with a particular focus on the 5 million people living in what is considered the world's greatest environmental disaster area, the Aral Sea area. Reference is also made to the high rate of TB in Russian prisons.

Reemergence of Infectious Disease in the Former Soviet Union

With the drastic economic, political, and environmental changes in the landscape of the FSU came a change in disease patterns in the last decade of the 20th century. Diseases that were well controlled, well hidden, or simply not prevalent during the Soviet period began to appear. The recent development of an HIV/AIDS epidemic in the Slavic states is an ominous precursor to similar developments in the Caucasus and Central Asia in the near future. From the start of the outbreak in Russia in 1987 until 1995, the total number of HIV-positive individuals officially registered was relatively small. During 1996 alone, however, 1,495 new infections were officially registered. In 1997, 4,337 new infections were registered of which 3,200 were among intravenous drug users. By the end of 1998, the total number of persons officially registered was more than 10,000, and by June 1999, the total had climbed to more than 14,000.

Because of possible inaccuracies in counting, however, it is possible that at the end of 1999 there are 100,000 to 200,000 persons with HIV in Russia alone. The socioeconomic upheaval in Russia and other countries of the FSU has seriously hampered the health system's ability to respond to this epidemic. The health system is overburdened and severely underfunded, resulting in material shortages and the nonpayment of salaries. Years of isolation from international research on HIV/AIDS, concomitant with the stigma associated with the disease, contributed to a basic lack of HIV/AIDS knowledge among health workers and the public.

The incidence of diphtheria has also skyrocketed in recent years. In 1980, the region accounted for less than 1 percent of diphtheria cases worldwide. By 1994, almost 90 percent of reported cases were occurring in the region, with more than 50,000 cases reported in 1995.

The incidence of malaria, which had been all but eradicated in the FSU, in the last few years has shown an alarming increase in the most southern states— from a few incidental and most likely imported cases of malaria in Tajikistan in the early 1990s, to almost 20,000 cases reported in 1998. In a region with a vast amount of stagnant water because of ineffective irrigation schemes and an entire generation of people with no experience with malaria prevention, a public health crisis is in the making as the malaria belt moves north.

It is TB, however, that typifies the threat that reemerging diseases can have on the FSU. The TB incidence rates in the FSU vary from country to country, with rates of anywhere from 50 per 100,000 population in Russia to a high of 300 per 100,000 population in the Aral Sea area of Central Asia. This represents more then a doubling of cases in less than 7 years. The prison population has an incidence 60 to 100 times higher than that among the civilian population. The uniqueness of the problem lies in the proportion of multidrug-resistant TB (MDR-TB) cases in civilian society, which is roughly 5 to 10 percent of all cases, and in the prison setting, where at least 20 percent of all patients have MDR-TB. These high rates of MDR-TB, in contrast to the rates in other regions of the world, reflect the breakdown of the political, economic, and health infrastructures in the region.

Political and Economic Causes of TB Reemergence

The Soviet Union had a very effective, albeit unsustainable, TB prevention and control infrastructure. With the break-up of the Soviet Union, however, the ensuing economic collapse, and the redirection of political priorities, the TB prevention infrastructure fell apart. The governments of the region and health care workers showed reluctance to adopt the WHO-developed directly observed treatment (short course) strategy (DOTS). In several countries, the old Soviet law, which outlawed the reporting and even the use of the word "epidemic," is still in the minds of health workers and politicians, even though it is not on the books. Such attitudes have slowed the reform of the TB prevention and control infrastructure.

Regional and other governments have shown a dangerous disregard for TB. TB is a disease that is either treated well, or not at all. The effect of the remnants of the old TB program is the development of MDR-TB. The drugs required to treat pansensitive TB cost roughly $15 to $40. The costs of drugs used to treat MDR-TB are 250 times more, and even then, cure rates reach only 50 percent. It has been estimated that $600 million would be required to cover 70 percent of the world TB cases with DOTS. Total international aid for TB in 1997 was a paltry $16 million. At present, however, MDR-TB has increased the transnational public health threat, and the costs associated with combating the disease cannot be met locally.

Directly associated with the economic collapse and the lack of political commitment is a long list of forces at play, and these are driving the TB epidemic in the FSU. They include the following:

• Lack of surveillance, monitoring, and program evaluation. The only way a reliable rate of TB can be determined is with a rigorous TB control program in place. This presents a paradox: the stronger the TB control program, the greater the chances that the incidence of TB is insignificant. Conversely, the time when monitoring is of utmost importance is precisely the time when epidemiological surveillance capacity is likely to be poor. Moreover, in the FSU an accurate denominator cannot be determined to arrive at an incidence rate because a census has not been taken since 1989 and millions of people have migrated throughout the region.

• Slowness in adapting new and effective protocols, such as DOTS. As of June 1998, within the five Central Asian countries, less than 2 percent of the estimated 50 million people were surveyed by DOTS. The longer this occurs, the greater the amplification of TB drug resistance, leading to the development of MDR-TB when DOTS is no longer effective. In addition, how likely is it that countries that have been slow in adopting DOTS will refer to DOTS Plus, a second-line drug treatment regimen for MDR-TB?

- Lack of drugs. The countries of Central Asia are not in a position to finance the three- to four-drug regimen associated with a DOTS program, let alone consider adding second-line drugs for the treatment of MDR-TB.
- Poor laboratory quality. The Soviet TB treatment protocol had an overreliance on X-rays for the diagnosis of TB, in contrast to a DOTS program, which primarily relies on sputum smear microscopy for the diagnosis of TB. Most laboratories that were once equipped with such diagnostic tools were underused and are now almost in a state of complete collapse, lacking even basic reagents. In all of Central Asia, it is safe to say that not one laboratory has the capacity to conduct culture and drug sensitivity testing for the 50 million people in the region, with a scarce few laboratories that can even perform simple diagnostic tests.
- Deteriorating physical infrastructure and logistics management. A cornerstone of the centralized economy in the FSU was the assignment of productive enterprises to various regions. When the FSU collapsed, the entire logistics chain broke as well. As a result, health care resources and logistics in Central Asia have been overlooked. It is common that facilities are not able to separate the infectious from the noninfectious patients, let alone provide a minimum level of hygiene. Moreover, the buildings are often cold during winter months and are dark and unventilated, providing an environment conducive to the spread of the disease.
- Lack of trained health workers. There is a generalized myth about an abundant supply of health practitioners in the FSU. Indeed, during the Soviet era, health care workers were numerous and well trained. In the Aral Sea area, not only has there been a significant exodus of trained staff because of the environmental disaster, placing a huge strain on the capacity of the health system, but the majority of health care workers who have remained in the region are nearing retirement and have had little to no upgrading of their skills. Given an average monthly salary of roughly $20, it is not surprising that few young people are entering the medical system, let alone dedicating their lives to TB—often literally, given nonexistent staff safety measures.
- Lack of financing and misdirected priorities. A cost-effectiveness study in Uzbekistan that compared the economic treatment costs of the traditional Soviet TB protocol and DOTS showed that if the government implemented DOTS, a savings of $5 million per year would be incurred. Once the epidemic was under control, the savings would continue to increase because of the immediate decrease in prevalence and the gradual decrease in incidence. Yet, there is still reliance on expensive mass screening programs using radiology.

Special Problems of the Prisons

Forty-two percent of all TB cases in Russia are among members of the prison population. Little is known about the prisoner infection rate in Central

Asia, but it is likely to be similar to, if not worse than that in Russia. Metaphorically, the Russian prison system is a petri dish that cultures various strains of the TB bacillus. Every year the system incarcerates 300,000 otherwise healthy Russians and releases another 300,000, most of whom will have been exposed to TB during their incarcerations. Among them, approximately 10 percent develop active disease and 80 percent carry the TB bacterium in a latent state; approximately 40 percent of all patients are exposed to MDR strains. The cause of high levels of drug resistance is the delay in the implementation of DOTS and the lack of prison reform. The crisis is almost at the point at which, unless second-line drugs are introduced in the prison system, the situation will never be controlled.

Role of Nongovernmental Organizations

To date few organizations have been active in TB control activities. NGOs can play a progressive role in this area by being proximate to the problem and, through advocacy, ensuring that the issue is placed on local, national, and international agendas. NGOs can develop pilot programs, conduct assessments, provide training, and contribute to the wider implementation of DOTS. NGO advocacy can be as straightforward and uncomplicated as the promotion of TB as a serious public health threat and DOTS as an effective way to control it. But without access to affordable and essential quality drugs and sustained financing, however, little progress can be made, particularly concerning MDR-TB.

NGOs can also advocate for increased activity in the private sector. Of the 1,233 drugs licensed worldwide between 1975 and 1997, only 13 were for tropical diseases and TB. Of those, two were slight modifications of existing drugs, two were produced for the U.S. military, and five were the outcomes of veterinary research. Drug companies, which spent a total of $40 billion on research in 1999, in two decades have developed only four medicines specifically for tropical diseases.

If NGOs become involved in the implementation of DOTS-based programs, they must be prepared to do it for the long run. It is unethical to enter a country, take away the country's existing tools for controlling TB (which are not fundamentally wrong, just inefficient and unsustainable), and leave before new methods have taken hold.

Pilot programs should balance the short-term objective of TB control in a specific area versus the long-term goal of complete DOTS coverage. Pilot programs should aim to develop momentum by reducing community stigmatization of TB, gaining patient and health worker confidence, and obtaining political commitment. Implementation of pilot programs is not the same as further extension of program coverage. The word "pilot" should not be used as a poor excuse for not wanting to accept responsibility for what happens next. Pilot programs should be monitored by using a set of assessment criteria to set the course for the full coverage of DOTS. These "DOTS-for-ALL" assess the following:

- documentation and the evaluation of the pilot phase and lessons learned,
- training requirements,
- laboratory capacity and quality,
- reliability and availability of epidemiological data,
- MDR,
- logistic capacity,
- whether donor and financial commitments are sustainable, and
- political commitment.

Conclusion

Although this discussion has concentrated particularly on TB as an example of an emerging and reemerging infectious disease, it highlights multiple concerns that apply equally to other infectious diseases in the FSU and surrounding regions. Nevertheless, TB exhibits several characteristics that make it one of the single largest health burdens in the region.

EUROPEAN RESPONSES TO EMERGING INFECTIONS AND THEIR POLICY IMPLICATIONS

Julius Weinberg, M.D.
Pro-Vice Chancellor (Research), School of Informatics,
City University, London, and Honorary Consultant Epidemiologist, Public
Health Laboratory Service, Communicable Disease Surveillance Centre, London

It is important when setting priorities for control of emerging and reemerging infectious diseases that one does not lose sight of the importance of controlling diseases that persist, for example, acute respiratory infection in children in the developing world.

The European Union (EU) has changed the environment for public health issues by creating a multinational geographical area within which people and goods move freely and by providing funds and the opportunity to share information so that an appropriate supranational response can be made. Although Europe does not face the same types of infectious disease problems found in Asia, Africa, and Latin America, it has a unique set of issues to contend with in the area of infectious diseases. For example, WHO has had to assist the countries of Central and Eastern Europe with the rebuilding of their communicable disease surveillance activities. The collapse of the previous regimes, military conflict, and the breakdown of public health measures has led to the recrudescence of some old problem diseases, in particular, diphtheria and TB, and has also led to anxieties about other diseases (e.g., typhus).

The movement of people around Europe has been associated with problems such as the resurgence of syphilis in Finland, importations of resistant TB into many countries, importation of resistant pneumococcus from Spain to Iceland, and the encroaching HIV/AIDS epidemic. The EU response has been to develop networks around specific agents, such as *Legionella* and *Salmonella*. The networks have facilitated rapid communication and response. For example, an outbreak of salmonella in the United Kingdom led to the identification of contaminated batches of a children's snack in several other European countries and the United States. Several outbreaks of legionellosis, which may not otherwise have been recognized, have been identified and controlled as a result of the timely pooling of data from a number of countries.

Antimicrobial resistance cannot be dealt with at the national level; it requires international collaboration. The European Antimicrobial Resistance Surveillance System (EARSS) is being developed. This will facilitate the sharing of methodology and data. As resistant organisms do not respect national boundaries, there will need to be collaboration of national and international efforts against resistance.

In addition to the disease- and organism-based networks, a number of infrastructure-related collaborations have been developed. The European Programme for Intervention Epidemiology Training (EPIET), which involves several EU countries in core training and exchanges, may provide the EU with the nucleus of a European system of trained and trainee epidemiologists who can provide support during international outbreaks. Other infrastructure developments include informatics programs and Worldwide web-based databases that will soon provide important information on laboratories within Europe that have the capacity to support and assist with investigations of certain outbreaks.

Critical aspects of international collaborations are establishing trust and harmonizing epidemiological and laboratory practices. One of the great successes of EntreNet, a network established to improve the prevention and control of human salmonellosis and other food-borne infections in European Union countries, has been the development of a Europe-wide typing system for *Salmonella enterica* serovar Enteritidis, a process that has resulted in the development of trust, collaboration, and exchange of materials. Conflicts can arise, however, around jurisdictions, costs, and international politics. Furthermore, countries have different traditions of accountability and data dissemination that must be acknowledged and considered. In addition, there may be conflicts with international agencies, such as the WHO, and with NGOs. The potential for disagreement must be recognized and dealt with early.

An important consideration in international collaborations is that national work always comes first, which can sometimes cause tensions and strains on resources, especially for smaller countries. On the positive side, collaborations can result in the sharing of good ideas. For example, in the United Kingdom a public education campaign that uses the character "Andy Biotic" aims to inform the general public about inappropriate antibiotic use. Similar campaigns are ongoing in Ireland and Sweden.

To develop consensus across diverse nationalities, a Delphi exercise was used to develop a plan on communicable disease surveillance at the European level. The plan was based on completion of a priority ranking of topics for collaboration by using the knowledge and experience of national experts in a consensus method adapted from the Delphi technique. By this technique, consensus is reached by means of questionnaires and feedback rounds circulated among a group of experts. The method retains anonymity and avoids the drawbacks of committee settings, such as domination or coalition. The exercise also tapped people's opinions about important mechanisms for collaboration, such as information exchange for early warnings and early detection through the pooling of data.

Such ranking exercises would yield different results in different regions of the world or if, for example, the global burden of disease were a primary consideration. However, they have value in developing consensus and in generating outputs that can be used to plan future programs. For example, a list of priorities was submitted as expert advice to the European Commission. Influenza was identified as a high priority for international surveillance, as was acute poliomyclitis, antimicrobial resistance, and cholera.

References

Aviles, G., Rangen, G., Vorndam, V., Briones, A., Baroni, P., Enria, D., and M.S. Sabattini. 1999. Dengue reemergence in Argentina. *Emerging Infectious Diseases* 5:575–578.

Cardosa, M.J., Krishnan, S., Tio, P.H., Perera, D., and S.C. Wong. 1999. Isolation of subgenus B adenovirus during a fatal outbreak of enterovirus 71-associated hand, foot, and mouth disease in Sibu, Sarawak. *Lancet* 354:987–991.

Chua, K.B., Goh, K.J., Wong, K.T., Kamarulzaman, A., Tan, B.S., Ksiazek, T.G., Zaki, S.R., Paul, G., Lam, S.K., and C.T. Tan. 1999. Fatal encephalitis due to Nipah virus among pig-farmers in Malaysia. *Lancet* 354:1257–1259.

Enria D., Padula, P., Segura, E.L., Pini, N., Edelstein, A, Riva Posse, C., and M.C. Weissenbacher. 1996. Hantavirus pulmonary syndrome in Argentina. Possibility of person to person transmission. *Medicina (Buenos Aires.)* 56:709–711.

Enria, D.A., Briggiler, A.M., and M.R. Feuilade. 1998. An overview of the epidemiological, ecological and preventive hallmarks of Argentine hemorrhagic fever (Junin virus). *Bulletin de l'Institut Pasteur* 96:103–114.

Fleming, D.M., and K.W. Cross. 1993. Respiratory syncytial virus or influenza? *Lancet* 342:1507–1510.

Huang, C.C., Liu, C.C., Chang, Y.C., Chen, C.Y., Wang, S.T., and T.F. Yeh. 1999. Neurological complications in children with enterovirus 71 infection. *New England Journal of Medicine* 341:936–942.

IOM (Institute of Medicine). 1988. *The Future of Public Health*. Washington, D.C.: National Academy Press.

IOM. 1992. *Emerging Infections: Microbial Threats to Health in the United States*. Washington, D.C.: National Academy Press.

IOM. 1997. *Orphans and Incentives: Developing Technologies to Address Emerging Infections*. Workshop Report. Washington, D.C.: National Academy Press.

IOM. 1998. *Antimicrobial Resistance: Issues and Options*. Workshop Report. Washington, D.C.: National Academy Press.

IOM. 2000a. *Managed Care Systems and Emerging Infections: Challenges and Opportunites for Strengthening Surveillance, Research, and Prevention. Workshop Summary*. Washington, D.C.: National Academy Press.

IOM. 2000b. *Public Health Systems and Emerging Infections: Assessing the Capabilities of the Public and Private Sectors*. Workshop Summary. Washington, D.C.: National Academy Press.

Kantor, I., Latini, O., and L. Barrera. 1998. La resistencia (y multirresistencia) a los medicamentos antituberculosos en Argentina y en otros países de América Latina. *Medicina (Buenos Aires)* 58:202–208.

Lam, S.K.1998. Emerging infectious diseases—Southeast Asia. *Emerging Infectious Diseases* 4:145–147.

Lucy, C.S., Lum, K.T., Wong, S.K., Lam, S.K., Chua, K.B., Goh, A.Y., Lim, W.L., Ong, B.B., Paul, G., AbuBaker, S., and M. Lambert. 1998. Fatal enterovirus 71 encephalomyelitis. *Journal of Pediatrics* 133:795–798.

Ministry of Health and Social Welfare of Argentina. July 1999. *Boletín sobre el SIDA en la Argentina VI*.

Padula, P.J., Edelstein, A., Miguel, S.D.L., López, N.M., Rossi, C.M., and R.D. Rabinovich. 1998. Hantavirus pulmonary syndrome outbreak in Argentina: molecular evidence for person-to-person transmission of Andes virus. *Virology* 241:323–330.

Rivas, M., Voyer, L.E., Tous, M., de Mena, M.F., Leardini, N., Wainsztein, R., Callejo, R., Quadri, B., and V. Prado. 1994. Verotoxin-producing "Escherichia coli" infection in household contacts of children with the hemolytic-uremic syndrome. In: *Recent Advances in Verocytotoxin-Producing "Escherichia coli" Infections*. M.A. Karmali and A.G. Goglio (eds.), pp. 49–52, Amsterdam: Elsevier Science B.V.

Rossi, A., Galas, M., Tokumoto, M., Guelfand, L., and H. Lopardo. 1999. Grupo colaborativo WHONET-Argentina. Actividad in vitro de trovafloxacina, otras fluoroquinolonas y de diferentes antimicrobianos frente a aislamientos clínicos. *Medicina (Buenos Aires)* 59(Suppl. I):8–16.

Sosa Estani, S., Campanini, A., Sinagra, A., Luna, C., Peralta, M., Coutada, V., Medina, L., Riarte, A., Salomón, O.D., Gomez, A., and E.L. Segura. 1998. Caracteristicas clínicas y diagnóstico de la Leishmaniasis mucocutanea en pacientes de un área endémica de Salta, Argentina. *Medicina (Buenos Aires)*, 58:685–691.

Varela, P., Pollevick, G.D., Rivas, M., Chinen, I., Binsztein, N., Frasch, A.C., and R.A. Ugalde. 1994. Direct detection of *Vibrio cholerae* in stool samples. *Journal of Clinical Microbiology* 32:1246–1248.

Weissenbacher, M.C., Guerrero, L.B., Help G., and A.S. Parodo. 1969. Inmunizacion contra la Fiebre Hemorragica Argentina con una cepa atenuada de Virus Junin. III Reacciones serologicas en voluntarios. *Medicina (Buenos Aires)* 29:88–92.

Wells, R.M., Sosa Estani, S., Yadon, Z.E., Enría, D., Padula, P., Pini, N., Mills, J.N., Peters, C.J., and E.L. Segura. 1997. An unusual hantavirus outbreak in Southern Argentina: Person-to-person transmission? *Emerging Infectious Diseases* 3:171–174.

Wong, K.T., Chua, K.B., and S.K. Lam. 1999. Immunohistochemical detection of infected neurons as a rapid diagnosis of enterovirus 71 encephalomyelitis. *Annals of Neurology* 45:271–272.

World Health Organization. 1999. *Report on Infectious Diseases: Removing obstacles to Healthy Development*. WHO/CDS/99.1. Geneva.

APPENDIX A

Glossary and Acronyms

This glossary is intended to define terms commonly encountered throughout this report as well as some terms that are commonly used in the public health arena. This glossary is not all inclusive. New terms and new usages of existing terms will emerge with time and with advances in technology. The definitions for the terms presented here were compiled from a multitude of sources, which are listed at the end of the glossary.

AAFP (American Academy of Family Physicians): A national, nonprofit medical association founded to promote and maintain high-quality standards for family doctors who are providing continuing comprehensive health care to the public (www.aafp.org).

AAMC (Association of American Medical Colleges): A nonprofit association whose purpose is to improve the nation's health (www.aamc.org).

AHCPR (Agency for Health Care Policy and Research): An agency of the U.S. Department of Health and Human Services that is charged with supporting research designed to improve the quality of health care, reduce its cost, and broaden access to essential services (www.ahcpr.gov).

AHCs (Academic Health Centers): Academic health centers, or AHCs, consist of health care institutions that are owned by or closely affiliated with a university or medical school. AHCs also have at least one additional health professional program and are engaged in undergraduate and graduate medical education, biomedical research, and delivery of patient care.

Antibiotic: Class of substances or chemicals that can kill or inhibit the growth of bacteria. Originally antibiotics were derived from natural sources (e.g., penicillin was derived from molds), but many currently used antibiotics are semisynthetic and are modified by the addition of artificial chemical components.

Antibiotic resistance: Property of bacteria that confers the capacity to inactivate or exclude antibiotics or a mechanism that blocks the inhibitory or killing effects of antibiotics.

Antimicrobial agents: Class of substances that can destroy or inhibit the growth of pathogenic groups of microorganisms, including bacteria, viruses, parasites, and fungi.

ASM (American Society for Microbiology): The oldest and largest membership organization in the world devoted to a single life science. ASM represents 24 disciplines of microbiological specializations plus a division for microbiology educators (www.asmusa.org).

Bacteria: Microscopic, single-celled organisms that have some biochemical and structural features different from those of animal and plant cells.

Basic research: Fundamental, theoretical, or experimental investigation to advance scientific knowledge, with immediate practical application not being a direct objective.

Benchmark: For a particular indicator or performance goal, the industry measure of best performance. The benchmarking process identifies the best performance in the industry (health care or non-health care) for a particular process or outcome, determines how that performance is achieved, and applies the lessons learned to improve performance.

Breteau Index: A derived measurement of the density of larval populations of *Aedes aegypti* mosquitoes used in vector-borne disease epidemiology (such as dengue and yellow fever). Generally, the higher the value of the Breteau Index the greater the relative abundance of *A. aegypti*, which results in an increased risk of vector-borne disease transmission in an area during a specified period of time.

Broad-spectrum antibiotic: An antibiotic effective against a large number of bacterial species. It generally describes antibiotics effective against both gram-positive and gram-negative classes of bacteria.

CDC (Centers for Disease Control and Prevention): A public health agency of the U.S. Department of Health and Human Services whose mission is to promote health and quality of life by preventing and controlling disease, injury, and disability (www.cdc.gov).

Clinical practice guidelines: Systematically developed statements that assist practitioners and patients with decision making about appropriate health care for specific clinical circumstances.

Clinical research: Investigations aimed at translating basic, fundamental science into medical practice.

Clinical trials: As used in this report, research with human volunteers to establish the safety and efficacy of a drug, such as an antibiotic or a vaccine.

Clinicians: One qualified or engaged in the clinical practice of medicine, psychiatry, or psychology, as distinguished from one specializing in laboratory or research techniques in the same fields.

DHHS (U.S. Department of Health and Human Services): The U.S. government's principal agency for protecting the health of all Americans and providing essential human services, especially for those who are least able to help themselves (www.os.dhhs.gov).

Directly Observed Treatment Short-course (DOTS): A short-course chemotherapy regimen for the treatment of tuberculosis (TB) that lasts 6 to 8 months and uses a combination of powerful anti-TB drugs under the direct observation by someone who is willing, trained, responsible, acceptable to the patient, and accountable to the TB control services.

Disease: The condition in which the functioning of the body or a part of the body is interfered with or damaged. In a person with an infectious disease, the infectious agent that has entered the body causes it to function abnormally in some way or ways. The type of abnormal functioning that occurs is the disease. Usually the body will show some signs and symptoms of the problems that it is having with functioning. Disease should not be confused with infection.

Emerging infections: Any infectious disease that has come to medical attention within the last two decades or for which there is a threat that its prevalence will increase in the near future (IOM, 1992). Many times, such diseases exist in nature as zoonoses and emerge as human pathogens only when humans come into contact with a formerly isolated animal population, such as monkeys in a rain forest that are no longer isolated because of deforestation. Drug-resistant organisms could also be included as the cause of emerging infections since they exist because of human influence. Some recent examples of agents responsible for emerging infections include human immunodeficiency virus, Ebola virus, and multidrug-resistant *Mycobacterium tuberculosis*.

Encephalitis: An acute inflammatory disease of the brain due to direct viral invasion or to hypersensitivity initiated by a virus or other foreign protein.

Endemic: Disease that is present in a community or common among a group of people; said of a disease continually prevailing in a region.

Enzootic: A disease of low morbidity that is constantly present in an animal community.

EPED: Epidemiologist's Editor as a general word processor.

EPIAIDS: A programmable word processing program within the Epidemiologist's Editor (EPED) word processor. EPIAIDS programs are provided to guide one through tutorials on the use of EPED and other programs and to assist in constructing memoranda, questionnaires, and epidemiological study designs.

Epizootic: A disease of high morbidity that is only occasionally present in an animal community.

Etiology: Science and study of the causes of diseases and their mode of operation.

FDA (U.S. Food and Drug Administration): A public health agency of the U.S. Department of Health and Human Services charged with protecting American consumers by enforcing the Federal Food, Drug, and Cosmetic Act and several related health laws (www.fda.gov).

FIC (Fogarty International Center): is a component of the international research effort of the National Institutes of Health (NIH). The FIC is responsible for advancing health through international scientific cooperation. FIC assumed a leadership role in formulating and implementing NIH biomedical research and policy in priority global health areas and in developing human capital and building research capacity in the poorest nations of the world, where the need is the greatest.

FoodNet: A set of activities designed to determine and monitor the burden of foodborne diseases and improve understanding of the proportion of foodborne diseases attributable to various pathogens. It is an example of population-based surveillance in the emerging infections programs.

Formulary: List of drugs approved for the treatment of various medical indications. It was originally created as a cost-control measure, but it has been used more recently to guide the use of antibiotics on the basis of information about resistance patterns.

HMO (health maintenance organization): A health care service plan that requires its subscriber members, except in a medical emergency, to use the services of designated physicians, hospitals, or other providers of medical care. HMOs typically use a capitation payment system that rewards providers for cost-effective management of patients.

Immunogenicity: The property that endows a substance with the capacity to provoke an immune response or the degree to which a substance possesses this property.

Incidence: The frequency of new occurrences of disease within a defined time interval. Incidence rate is the number of new cases of a specified disease divided by the number of people in a population over a specified period of time, usually 1 year.

Infection: The invasion of the body or a part of the body by a pathogenic agent, such as a microoganism or virus. Under favorable conditions the agent develops or multiplies, the results of which may produce injurious effects. Infection should not be confused with disease.

Invasive isolates: A genetically homologous culture of a microorganism or virus that is capable of invading or penetrating the body or a part of the body.

MCO (managed care organization): An organization that arranges for health care delivery and financing and that is designed to provide appropriate, effective, and efficient health care through organized relationships with providers. Includes formal programs for ongoing quality assurance and utilization review, financial incentives for covered members to use the plan's providers, and financial incentives for providers to contain costs. Managed care plans vary greatly in the degree to which benefit coverage is offered, and monitored and also the degree to which benefits are conditioned on the basis of the meeting of certain criteria by the subscriber member and the member's primary care physician.

Meningitis: Inflammation of the membranes of the spinal cord or brain as a result of an infection of the fluid of a person's spinal cord and the fluid that surrounds the brain. Sometimes referred to as spinal meningitis. Meningitis is usually caused by a viral or bacterial infection.

MIC (minimum inhibitory concentration): The lowest antibiotic concentration that prevents bacterial growth.

MRSA (methicillin-resistant *Staphylococcus aureus*): In strict terms, a *Staphylococcus aureus* strain resistant to the antibiotic methicillin. In practice, MRSA strains are generally resistant to many antibiotics, and some are resistant to all antibiotics except vancomycin, such that the acronym is now generally used to mean "multidrug-resistant *S. aureus.*"

NCID (National Center for Infectious Diseases): The division of the Centers for Disease Control and Prevention whose mission is to prevent illness, disability, and death caused by infectious diseases in the United States and around the world. NCID accomplishes its mission by conducting surveillance, epidemic investigations, epidemiological and laboratory research, training, and public education programs to develop, evaluate, and promote prevention and control strategies for infectious diseases (www.cdc.gov/ncidod/ncid.htm).

NIAID (National Institute of Allergy and Infectious Diseases): A division of the National Institutes of Health that provides the major support for scientists conducting research aimed at developing better ways to diagnose, treat, and prevent the many infectious, immunological, and allergenic diseases that afflict people worldwide (www.niaid.nih.gov).

NIH (National Institutes of Health): A public health agency of the U.S. Department of Health and Human Services whose goal is to acquire new knowledge to help prevent, detect, diagnose, and treat disease and disability, from the rarest genetic disorder to the common cold (www.nih.gov).

Nosocomial infection: An infection that is acquired during hospitalization but that was neither present nor incubating at the time of hospital admission, unless it is related to a prior hospitalization, and that may become clinically manifest after discharge from the hospital.

Outpatient services: Medical and other health care services not requiring hospitalization. These services may be provided by a hospital or other qualified facility or supplier, such as mental health clinics, rural health clinics, mobile X-ray units, or freestanding dialysis units. Such services include outpatient physical therapy services, diagnostic X-ray and laboratory tests, and radiation therapy.

PA (Program Announcement): A public announcement describing the goals and scope of a proposed scientific project awaiting approval from a specific scientific organization.

Primary care: Basic or general health care, traditionally provided by family practice, pediatric, and internal medicine physicians.

Prophylactic antibiotics: Antibiotics that are administered before evidence of infection with the intention of warding off disease.

Public Health Service Act of 1944: An act to consolidate and revise the laws relating to the U.S. Public Health Service.

Sepsis: The pathological condition that results from the presence of pathogenic microorganisms or their toxins in blood or other tissues.

SSS (Sentinel Surveillance Systems): A type of surveillance that relies on reports of cases of disease whose occurrence suggests that the quality of preventive or therapeutic medical care needs to be improved.

Surveillance systems: Used in this report to refer to data collection and record-keeping to track the emergence and spread of disease-causing organisms such as antibiotic-resistant bacteria.

Sylvatic disease: An infectious disease spread among wild animals living in forests.

Vaccine: A preparation of living, attenuated, or killed bacteria or viruses, fractions thereof, or synthesized or recombinant antigens identical or similar to those found in the disease-causing organisms that is administered to raise immunity to a particular microorganism.

Zoonotic disease or infection: An infection or infectious disease that may be transmitted from vertebrate animals (e.g., a rodent) to humans.

Definitions for this glossary were compiled from the following sources:

American Academy of Family Physicians, Federal Advocacy Sites (date of last update: January 17, 2000). Available at: www.aafp.org/fpnet/guide/append_d.html

American Academy of Pediatrics (date of last update: March 26, 1999). Available at: www.aap.org/advocacy/washing/fedinfo.htm.

American Association of Health Plans, Network-Based Health Plans Definitions (date of last update: July 19, 1998). Available at: www.aahp.org/menus/index1.cfm.

American College of Obstetricians and Gynecologists: Women's Health Care Physicians. Available at: www.acog.com.

American Medical Association. *Manual of Style*, 9th ed. Chicago: American Medical Association, 1998.

Association of American Medical Colleges (date of last update: December 7, 1999). Available at: www.aamc.org.

Centers for Disease Control and Prevention. Available at: www.cdc.gov.

Dorland's Illustrated Medical Dictionary, 28th ed. Philadelphia: The W. B. Saunders Co., 1994.

Health Care Quality Glossary (date of last update: February 8, 2000) Overview. The Russia-United States of America Joint Commission on Economic and Technological Cooperation, The Health Committee, Access to Quality Health Care, 1999. Agency for Health Care Policy and Research, Rockville, Md. Available at: www.ahrq.gov/ qual/hcqgloss.htm.

Institute of Medicine. *Orphans and Incentives: Developing Technologies to Address Emerging Infections.* Workshop Report. Washington, D.C.: National Academy Press, 1997.

Institute of Medicine. *Antimicrobial Resistance: Issues and Options.* Workshop Report. Washington, D.C.: National Academy Press, 1998.

Institute of Medicine. *Managed Care Systems and Emerging Infections: Challenges and Opportunities for Strengthening Surveillance, Research, and Prevention. Workshop Summary.* Washington, D.C.: National Academy Press, 2000.

McGraw-Hill Dictionary of Scientific and Technical Terms, 5th ed. Washington, D.C.: McGraw-Hill, Inc., 1994.

Medline Plus (date of last update: May 3, 2000). Available at: www.nlm.nih.gov/medlineplus.

National Cancer Institute. Available at: www.nci.nih.gov.

National Center for Infectious Diseases (date of last update: May 3, 2000). Available at: www.cdc.gov/ncidod/index.htm.

National Human Genome Research Institute, Glossary of Genetic Terms (date of last update: December 29, 1999). Available at: www.nhgri.nih.gov/DIR/VIP/Glossary.

National Institute of Allergy and Infectious Diseases (date of last update: March 10, 1999). Available at: www.niaid.nih.gov.

National Institutes of Health. Available at: www.nih.gov.

OneLook Dictionaries. Available at: www.onelook.com.

U.S. Department of Health and Human Services. Available at: www.os.dhhs. gov.

U.S. Food and Drug Administration. Available at: www.fda.gov.

Webster's Third New International Dictionary. Springfield, Mass.: Merriam-Webster, Inc., 1986.

APPENDIX B

Workshop Agenda

 Institute of Medicine
The National Academies

FORUM ON EMERGING INFECTIONS
International Aspects of Emerging Infections
National Academy of Sciences Auditorium
2101 Constitution Avenue, N.W., Washington, D.C.

THURSDAY, 28 OCTOBER 1999

8:30a.m.   **Welcome and Opening Remarks**
             Joshua Lederberg, *Chair*, Forum on Emerging Infections

8:45   **Keynote Address**
             David Heymann, Executive Director, Communicable
             Diseases, World Health Organization

9:30–12:45   **Emerging Infections in the Americas**
             Moderator: David Shlaes, *Forum Member*

9:30   **Emerging Infections in Colombia: A National Perspective**
             Jorge Boshell-Samper, Director General, Instituto Nacional de
             Salud, Colombia

10:00   **A National Strategy for Emerging Infectious Diseases:**
                   The Argentine Case of 1999
                   Elsa Segura, Director, Administración Nacional de
                   Laboratrios e Institutos de Salud, "Dr. Carlos G. Malbran,"
                   Argentina

10:30   **Break**

10:45   **The Response of the Pan American Health Organization**
                   (PAHO) to Emerging Infectious Diseases in Latin America
                   and the Caribbean
                   Francisco Pinheiro, Advisor on Viral Diseases, Division of
                   Disease Prevention and Control, Pan American Health
                   Organization

11:15   **Diagnosis, Epidemiological Surveillance, and Control**
                   Programs for Emerging and Reemerging Infectious
                   Diseases in Mexico
                   Ana Flisser, Director, National Institute for Epidemiological
                   Diagnosis and Reference (INDRE), Mexico

11:45   **PANEL DISCUSSION**
                   Panel Members
                   Speakers:
                   • Jorge Boshell-Samper
                   • Elsa Segura
                   • Francisco Pinheiro
                   • Ana Flisser

                   Invited Panelists:
                   • Steve Waterman, California Office of Border Health, CDC
                   • Robert Shope, University of Texas
                   • David Bell, Centers for Disease Control and Prevention
                   • Caryn Miller, USAID

12:45p.m.   **Lunch**

2:00–5:15   **EMERGING INFECTIONS IN AFRICA**
                   Moderator: Stephen Morse, *Forum Member*

| 2:00 | **Integrated Disease Surveillance and Epidemic Preparedness and Response in Africa** |
| | Bradley Perkins, Chief, Meningitis and Special Pathogens Branch, National Center for Infectious Diseases, Centers for Disease Control and Prevention, United States |

2:00   **Integrated Disease Surveillance and Epidemic Preparedness and Response in Africa**
Bradley Perkins, Chief, Meningitis and Special Pathogens Branch, National Center for Infectious Diseases, Centers for Disease Control and Prevention, United States

2:30   **Global Emerging Infections System (GEIS)**
Patrick W. Kelley, Director, Division of Preventive Medicine, Walter Reed Army Institute of Research, United States Army

3:00   **Emerging Infections in Africa: The WHO African Regional Office Response**

3:30   **Break**

4:15   Panel Discussion
Panel Members
Speakers:
- Bradley Perkins
- Patrick Kelley
- Antoine Kabore

Invited Panelists:
- Adel Mahmoud, Merck Vaccines
- Philip Coyne, World Bank
- Mary Ettling, USAID

5:15   **Adjournment**

FRIDAY, 29 OCTOBER 1999

8:30a.m.   **Opening Remarks**
Joshua Lederberg, *Chair*, Forum on Emerging Infections

8:45–12:00   **Emerging Infections in Asia and the Pacific**
Moderator: Gary Christopherson, *Forum Member*

8:45   **Emerging Infectious Diseases in Hong Kong and Their Public Health Significance**
Kwok Hang Mak, Department of Health, Hong Kong, China

9:15   **Emerging Diseases in the Australasian Region**
              John MacKenzie, Professor and Head, Department of
              Microbiology and Parasitology, The University of Queensland,
              Australia

9:45   **Past Review of Emerging Diseases of Thailand, Southeast
              Asia, and South Asia**

10:15   **International Smart Partnership in Emerging Diseases:
              Sense and Sensitivity**
              Lam Sai-Kit, Professor and Head, Department of Medical
              Microbiology, University of Malaya, Kuala Lumpur, Malaysia

10:45   **Break**

11:00   **Panel Discussion**
              Panel Members
              Speakers:
              • John MacKenzie
              • Lam Sai-Kit
              • K.H. Mak

              Invited Panelists:
              • Nancy Cox, Centers for Disease Control and Prevention
              • Ann Marie Kimball, University of Washington
              • Michael MacDonald, USAID-BASICS Project
              • Kaye Wachsmuth, USDA

12:00noon   **Lunch**

1:00–4:15   **EMERGING INFECTIONS IN EUROPE**
              Moderator: Renu Gupta, *Forum Member*

1:00   **Pandemic Strategic Planning**
              Jane Leese, Senior Medical Officer, Immunization Team,
              Department of Health, London, United Kingdom

1:30   **Emerging Infections in the Former Soviet Union, and the
              MSF International Campaign for Access to Drugs in
              Developing Countries**
              Ian Small, Director, Médicins sans Frontières, Tashkent,
              Uzbekistan

2:00   **European Responses to Emerging Infections and Their Policy Implications**
Julius Weinberg, Pro-Vice Chancellor (Research), School of Informatics, City University, London; Honorary Consultant Epidemiologist, Public Health Laboratory Service, Communicable Disease Surveillance Centre, London, United Kingdom

2:30   **Demonstration of the European Delphi Study**
Julius Weinberg, Pro-Vice Chancellor (Research), School of Informatics, City University, London; Honorary Consultant Epidemiologist, Public Health Laboratory Service, Communicable Disease Surveillance Centre, London, United Kingdom

3:00   **Break**

3:15   **PANEL DISCUSSION**
Panel Members
Speakers:
- Jane Leese
- Julius Weinberg
- Ian Small

Invited Panelists:
- Robert Steinglass, U.S. AID-BASICS Project
- David Fidler, University of Indiana
- James LeDuc, Centers for Disease Control and Prevention
- Mary Ann Micka, USAID
- Laura Efros, OSTP

4:15–5:30   **Summary and Concluding Remarks**
Moderator: Joshua Lederberg, *Chair*, Forum on Emerging Infections

4:15   **Summary and Discussion with Session Moderators**
Closing Remarks
Joshua Lederberg
Chair, Forum on Emerging Infections

5:30   **Adjournment**

APPENDIX C

Workshop Participants

Vincent I. Ahonkhai, M.D. [1]
Vice President and Director,
Anti-Infectives and Biologicals
SmithKline Beecham
    Corporation
1250 South Collegeville Road
P.O. Box 5089
Collegeville, PA 19426-0989

Allan N.D. Auclair, Ph.D. [4]
Senior Scientist, RAND
Environmental Science and Policy
    Center, Room 946
1333 H Street, N.W.
Washington, DC 20005-4707

David Bell, M.D. [3]
Assistant to the Director for Antimicro-
bial Resistance
National Center for Infectious Diseases
Centers for Disease Control and
    Prevention
1600 Clifton Road,
Mail Code C-12
Atlanta, GA 30333

Jorge Boshell-Samper M.D. [2]
General Director
Instituto Nacional de Salud
Avenida Eldorado, Carrera 50
A.A. 80080 Bogota, D.C.
COLOMBIA

NOTE: 1 = forum member, 2 = workshop speaker, 3 = workshop panelist, 4 = guest, and 5 = IOM staff.

Nancy Carter Foster, M.S.T.M. [1]
Director, Program for
    Emerging Infections and
    HIV/AIDS
U.S. Department of State
2201 C Street, N.W.
Washington, DC 20520

Gary Christopherson [1]
Principal Deputy Assistant
Secretary for Health Affairs
Department of Defense
The Pentagon, Room 3E 346
OASD (HA)
Washington, DC 20301-12000

Barney Cohen, Ph.D. [4]
Director, Committee on
    Population
2101 Constitution Ave., N.W.
Washington, DC 20418

Nancy Cox, Ph.D. [3]
Chief, Influenza Branch
Centers for Disease Control and
    Prevention
1600 Clifton Road
Building 7, Room 111
Mail Stop G 16
Atlanta, GA 30333

Philip Coyne, M.D. [3]
Tropical Medicine Consultant
World Bank Onchocerciasis
    Coordination Unit
Room J-8-029
1818 H Street, N.W.
Washington, DC 20433

Connie Davis [4]
Infectious Disease Advisor
Bureau for Africa
U.S. Agency for International
    Development
1325 G Street, N.W., Room 400
Washington, DC 20005

Jonathan R. Davis, Ph.D., M.S. [5]
Senior Study Director
Institute of Medicine
2101 Constitution Avenue, N.W.
Room FO3054
Washington, DC 20418

Madeline Drexler [4]
Journalist
197 Westminster Avenue
Watertown, MA 02472

Cedric DuMont M.D. [1]
Medical Director
Office of Medical Services
U.S. Department of State
Room L-209, SA-1
2401 E Street, N.W.
Washington, DC 20522-0102

Laura Efros, Ph.D. [3]
Senior Policy Advisor
White House Office of Science and
    Technology Policy
Old Executive Office Building
Room 494
Washington, DC 20502

Mary Ettling [3]
Technical Advisor
Bureau for Africa
US Agency for International
    Development
1325 G Street, N.W.
Room 447
Washington, DC 20005

David Fidler, J.D. [3]
Associate Professor
School of Law
Indiana University
211 South Indiana Avenue
Bloomington, IN 47405-1001

Ana Flisser, Ph.D. [2]
Director, National Institute for
    Epidemiological Diagnosis and
    Reference (INDRE)
Carpio 470
Colonia Santo Thomas
Mexico, D.F. 11340
MEXICO

Renu Gupta, M.D. [1]
Vice President, Medical, Safety and
Therapeutics Covance
210 Carnegie Center
Princeton, NJ 08540-6233

Leslie M. Hardy [4]
Special Assistant to the
Assistant Secretary for Planning
    and Evaluation DHHS/OASPE
200 Independence Avenue, S.W.
Room 405F
Washington, DC 20201

David Heymann, M.D. [2]
Executive Director
Communicable Diseases
World Health Organization
20, Avenue Appia
CH-1211 Geneva 27
SWITZERLAND

Lynn Holloway [4]
Assistant Director, GAO
International Relations and Trade
    Group,
National Security and International
    Affairs Division
441 G Street, N.W.
Washington, DC 20548

James M. Hughes, M.D. [1]
Assistant Surgeon General, and
    Director, National Center for
    Infectious Diseases
Centers for Disease Control and
    Prevention
1600 Clifton Road, N.E.,
Mailstop C-12
Atlanta, GA 30333

Jeffrey M. Johnston, M. D. [4]
Principal Clinical Program Head,
Infectious Diseases and Hepatitis
Glaxo Wellcome
Five Moore Drive
P.O. Box 13398
Research Triangle Park, NC
    27709-3398

Samuel L. Katz, M.D. [1]
Chairman of the Board
Burroughs Wellcome Fund, and
Wilburt C. Davison
Professor and Chairman Emeritus
Department of Pediatrics
Duke University Medical Center
Rm 1140A
Hospital South Yellow Zone
Trent Drive, Box 2925
Durham, NC 27710

Patrick W. Kelley, M.D., Dr.P.H. [1,2]
Colonel, U.S. Army,
Director, Department of Defense
    Global Emerging Infections
Surveillance and Response System
Division of Preventive Medicine
Walter Reed Army Institute of
Research, Bldg. 503
    Forest Glen Annex (Rm. 2S34)
Robert Grant Road
Silver Spring, MD 20910

Ann-Marie Kimball, M.D., M.P.H. [3]
Director, MPH Program and
    Community Medicine
School of Public Health and
    Community Medicine
Associate Professor of
    Epidemiology, Box 357660
University of Washington
Seattle, WA

**Lam Sai Kit, M.Sc., Ph.D.,
FRCPath, FRCP(Edin) FASc** [2]
Professor and Head
Department of Medical
    Microbiology
Faculty of Medicine
University of Malaya
50603 Kuala Lampur
MALAYSIA

Joshua Lederberg, Ph.D. [1]
Sackler Foundation Scholar
The Rockefeller University
1230 York Avenue
New York, NY 10021

James LeDuc, Ph.D. [3]
Associate Director for Global
    Health,
Centers for Disease Control and
    Prevention
1600 Clifton Road, NE-MSC12
Atlanta, GA 30333

Jane Leese, M.D. [2]
Senior Medical Officer
Immunization Team
Department of Health
Wellington House, Room 706
133-155 Waterloo Road
London SE1 8UG
UNITED KINGDOM

Carlos Lopez, Ph.D. [1]
Executive Director
Infectious Disease Research
Eli Lilly Research Laboratories
Lilly Corporate Center
Mail Drop 1705
Indianapolis, IN 46285-0438

Michael MacDonald, Sc.D. [3]
Technical Officer/Coordinator Malaria Activities, BASICS
1600 Wilson Boulevard,
Suite 300
Arlington, VA 22209

John S. Mackenzie, Ph.D. [2]
Department of Microbiology and
    Parasitology
The University of Queensland
Brisbane, Queensland 4072
AUSTRALIA

Adel Mahmoud, M.D., Ph.D. [3]
President, Merck Vaccines
Merck and Co., Inc.
One Merck Drive
Whitehouse Station, NJ 08889

Kwok Hang Mak, M.D. [2]
Consultant, Community Medicine,
Student Health Service
Department of Health
Government of The Hong Kong
    Special Adminstrative Region
4/F Lam Tin Polyclinic
99 Kai Tin Road Kwun Tonh
Kowloon
PEOPLE'S REPUBLIC OF
CHINA

Robert McCreight, Ph.D. [4]
Bureau of Intelligence and
    Research
Office of Research
US Department of State
2201 C Street, N.W.
Washington, DC 20520

Mary Ann Micka, Ph.D. [3]
Bureau for Europe and Eurasia
U.S. Agency for International
    Development
1300 Pennsylvania Avenue, N.W.
 Room 5.10-096
Washington, DC 20523-5100

Caryn Miller, Ph.D.[3]
U.S. Agency for International
    Development
1300 Pennsylvania Avenue, N.W.
Room 6.07.031
Washington, DC 20523

Nancy B. Mock, Dr.P.H. [4]
Director and Associate Professor of
    International Health
Tulane University
1440 Canal Street, Suite 2200
New Orleans, LA 70112

Roscoe M. Moore, Jr., M.D. [4]
Assistant Surgeon General
U.S. Public Health Service,
Department of Health and Human
    Services
5600 Fishers Lane, Room 18-87
Parklawn Building
Rockville, MD 20857

Stephen S. Morse, Ph.D. [1]
Professor of Epidemiology
Columbia University School of
    Public Health
600 West 168th Street
New York, NY 10032

Stuart L. Nightingale, M.D.[4]
Associate Commissioner for Health
    Affairs
Food and Drug Administration
Department of Health and Human
    Services
Parklawn Building, Room 15-36
5600 Fishers Lane
Rockville, MD 20857

Vivian P. Nolan [5]
Research Associate
Institute of Medicine
2101 Constitution Avenue, N.W.
Washington, DC 20418

Bradley A. Perkins, M.D. [2]
Chief, Meningitis and Special
    Pathogens Branch
Centers for Disease Control and
    Prevention
1600 Clifton Road
Building 1, Room 4055
Mail Stop C 09
Atlanta, GA 30333

Francisco Pinheiro, M.D. [2]
Advisor on Viral Diseases
Program of Communicable
    Diseases, Division of Disease
    Prevention and Control
Pan American Health Organization
525 23rd Street, N.W.
Washington, DC 20037-2895

Guénaël Rodier, M.D. [2]
Chief, Epidemiological
    Surveillance and Epidemic
    Response (EMC)
World Health Organization
20, Avenue Appia
CH-1211 Geneva 27
SWITZERLAND

Gary Roselle, M.D. [1]
Program Director for
Infectious Disease
Department of Veterans
Affairs
3200 Vine Street (111)
Cincinnati, OH 45220

Elsa L. Segura, Ph.D. [2]
Researcher of CONICET and of
    Administración Nacional de
    Laboratorios e Institutos
    de Salud "Dr. Carlos G.
    Malbrán"
Ave. Paseo Colón 568
1063 Buenos Aires
ARGENTINA

David M. Shlaes, M.D., Ph.D. [1]
Vice President,
Infectious Disease Research
Wyeth-Ayerst Research
401 N. Middletown Road
Pearl River, NY 10965

Robert E. Shope, M.D. [3]
Professor of Pathology
Department of Pathology
University of Texas Medical
    Branch
301 University Boulevard
Galveston, TX 77555-0609

Ian B. Small, M.A. [2]
Head of Mission
Médecins sans Frontières
PO Box 333
700 000 Tashkent
UZBEKISTAN

Robert Steinglass [3]
BASICS
1600 Wilson Boulevard,
Suite 300
Arlington, VA 22209

Nelle Temple-Brown, Ph.D. [4]
External Relations Officer
World Health Organization
1775 K St., N.W.
Suite 430
Washington, DC 20006

Juli Trtanj [4]
International Development
    Specialist,
UCAR Joint Office for Science
    Support
NOAA Office of Global Programs
1100 Wayne Avenue, Suite 1225
Silver Spring, MD 20910-5603

Kaye Wachsmuth, Ph.D. [3]
Deputy Administrator
Office of Public Health and
    Science FSIS/USDA
Room 341-E Whitten Building
1400 Independence Ave., S.W.
Washington, DC 20250-3700

Tessa Walters, M.D. [4]
Science Fellow
Center for International
    Security and Cooperation
Stanford University
Encina Hall
Stanford, CA 94305-6165

Steve Waterman, M.D., Ph.D. [3]
Senior Medical Epidemiologist
CDC Division of Quarantine
California Office of Border Health
1360 Plum Street
San Diego, CA 92106

Julius Weinberg, Ph.D. [2]
Professor, Pro-Vice Chancellor
    (Research) School of
    Informatics
City University
Northampton Square
London EC1V OHB
UNITED KINGDOM

APPENDIX D

Forum Member and Staff Biographies

FORUM MEMBERS

JOSHUA LEDERBERG, Ph.D., is Professor emeritus of molecular genetics and informatics and Sackler Foundation Scholar at The Rockefeller University, New York, New York. His lifelong research, for which he received the Nobel Prize in 1958, has been in genetic structure and function in microorganisms. He has a keen interest in international health and was cochair of a previous Institute of Medicine committee, the Committee on Emerging Microbial Threats to Health (1990–1992). He has been a member of the National Academy of Sciences since 1957 and is a charter member of the Institute of Medicine. Dr. Lederberg is the chair of the Forum on Emerging Infections.

VINCENT AHONKHAI, M.D., is Vice President and Director at SmithKline Beecham Pharmaceuticals and is responsible for clinical research and development and medical affairs in anti-infectives and biologicals in North America. He has held this position since 1995, overseeing a product portfolio that includes antibiotics, antivirals, and vaccines. After completing medical school and internships in Nigeria, Dr. Ahonkhai obtained additional training in pediatric residency, followed by a fellowship in infectious diseases in adults and pediatrics at the State University of New York–Downstate Medical Center, Brooklyn, from 1975 to 1980. He then joined the faculty as Assistant Professor, Department of Pediatrics. In 1982, Dr. Ahonkhai started his pharmaceutical industry career as Associate Director, Infectious Diseases, at Merck, where he rose to the director level. Subsequently, he moved to the Robert Wood Johnson Pharmaceutical Research Institute, where he served first as Head of Infectious Diseases and later as Executive Director, Dermatology and Wound Healing. Dr. Ahonkhai is board certified in pediatrics and is a long-standing member and fellow of several professional organizations including the American Medical Association, National Medical Association, American Society for Microbiology, Infectious Diseases Society of America (fellow), Pediatric Infectious Diseases Society, and American Academy of Pharmaceutical Physicians (Vice President, Membership Development Committee, and board member).

STEVEN J. BRICKNER, Ph.D., is Manager of Medicinal Chemistry at Pfizer Central Research, where he leads a team of medicinal chemists that is focused on the discovery and development of new antibacterial agents designed to meet the growing problems with resistance. He has more than 15 years of pharmaceutical industrial research experience, all directed at the discovery of novel antibiotics. Before joining Pfizer, he led a team that discovered and developed linezolid, the first oxazolidinone to undergo phase III clinical evaluation. Dr. Brickner is recognized as a world expert on this new class of antibacterial agents.

GAIL H. CASSELL, Ph.D., is Vice President, Infectious Diseases Research, Drug Discovery Research, and Clinical Investigation, at Eli Lilly & Company. Previously, she was the Charles H. McCauley Professor and (since 1987) Chair, Department of Microbiology, University of Alabama Schools of Medicine and Dentistry at Birmingham, a department which, under her leadership, has ranked first in research funding from the National Institutes of Health since 1989. She is a member of the Director's Advisory Committee of the national Centers for Disease Control and Prevention. Dr. Cassell is past president of the American Society for Microbiology, a former member of the National Institutes of Health Director's Advisory Committee, and a former member of the Advisory Council of the National Institute of Allergy and Infectious Diseases. She has also served as an advisor on infectious diseases and indirect costs of research to the White House Office on Science and Technology and was previously Chair of the Board of Scientific Councelors of the National Center for Infectious Diseases, Centers for Disease Control and Prevention. Dr. Cassell served 8 years on the Bacteriology-Mycology-II Study Section and served as its chair for 3 years. She serves on the editorial boards of several prestigious scientific journals and has authored more than 250 articles and book chapters. She has been intimately involved in the establishment of science policy and legislation related to biomedical research and public health. Dr. Cassell has received several national and international awards and an honorary degree for her research on infectious diseases.

GARY CHRISTOPHERSON, is Senior Adviser for Force Health Protection at the U.S. Department of Defense, Reserve Affairs. Previously, as Principal Deputy Assistant Secretary of Defense for Health Affairs, he managed policy, the Defense Health Program budget, and performance for the Military Health System, including the $16 billion TRICARE health care system and force health protection. In that role, he also launched the U.S. Department of State's infectious disease surveillance and response system and served as cochair on the White House's Infectious Disease Surveillance and Response Subcommittee. He has also been a key figure in the Department's Force Health Protection Initiative against anthrax. In early 1998, he served as the Acting Assistant Secretary of Defense for Health Affairs. Joining the U.S. Department of Defense in 1994, he has served as Health Affairs' Acting Principal Deputy Assistant Secretary and Senior Adviser, where he provided advice on a wide range of health issues and managed the relationships with the White House and other federal agencies. Previously, he served 2 years (1992–1994) with the Office of Presidential Personnel at the White House and the Presidential Transition Office. As Associate Director, he managed the President's appointments (PAS/PA/SES level) to the U.S. Departments of Health and Human Services and Defense as well as 10 other departments. Before that he served in a number of senior health positions with the Congress and with public and private public health agencies.

GORDON DeFRIESE, Ph.D., is Professor of Social Medicine, Epidemiology, and Health Policy and Administration and Director of the Cecil G. Sheps Center for Health Services Research at the University of North Carolina at Chapel Hill. He received his Ph.D. from the University of Kentucky College of Medicine. Some of his research interests are in the areas of health promotion and disease prevention, medical sociology, primary health care, rural health care, cost-benefit analysis, and cost-effectiveness. He is a member of the Global Advisory Group on Health Systems Research of the World Health Organization in Geneva, Switzerland, past president of the Association for Health Services Research and the Foundation for Health Services Research, and a fellow of the New York Academy of Medicine. He is founder of the Partnership for Prevention, a coalition of private-sector business and industry organizations, voluntary health organizations, and state and federal public health agencies based in Washington, D.C., that have joined together to work toward the elevation of disease prevention among the nation's health policy priorities.

CEDRIC E. DUMONT, M.D., is Medical Director for the Office of Medical Services (MED) at the U.S. Department of State. Dr. Dumont graduated from Columbia University with a B.A. in 1975 and obtained his medical degree from Tufts University School of Medicine in 1980. Dr. Dumont is a board-certified internist with subspecialty training in infectious diseases. He completed his internal medicine residency in 1983 and infectious diseases fellowship in 1988 at Georgetown University Hospital in Washington, D.C. Dr. Dumont has been a medical practitioner for more than 19 years, 2 of which included service in the Peace Corps. Since joining the U.S. Department of State in 1990, he has had substantial experience overseas in Dakar, Senegal; Bamako, Mali; Kinshasa, Zaire; and Brazzaville, Congo. For the past 3 years, as the Medical Director for the U.S. Department of State, Dr. Dumont has promoted the health of all United States Government employees serving overseas by encouraging their participation in a comprehensive health maintenance program and by facilitating their access to high-quality medical care. Dr. Dumont is a very strong supporter of the professional development and advancement of MED's highly qualified professional staff. In addition, he has supported and encouraged the use of an electronic medical record, which will be able to monitor the health of all its beneficiaries, not only during a specific assignment but also throughout their career in the Foreign Service.

JESSE GOODMAN, M.D., M.P.H., was Professor of Medicine and Chief of Infectious Diseases at the University of Minnesota and is now serving as Deputy Medical Director for the U.S. Food and Drug Administration's (FDA's) Center for Biologics Evaluation and Research, where he is active in a broad range of policy issues. After joining the FDA Commissioner's office, he has worked closely with several centers and helped coordinate FDA's response to the antimicrobial resistance problem. He is also cochair of a recently formed federal interagency task force to develop a national action plan on antimicrobial resistance. He graduated from Harvard College and attended the Albert Einstein College of Medicine, followed by internal medicine, hematology, oncology, and infectious diseases training at the University of Pennsylvania and University of California, Los Angeles, where he was also Chief Medical Resident. He received his master's of public health degree from the University of Minnesota. In recent years, his laboratory's research has focused on the molecular pathogenesis of tick-borne diseases. His laboratory isolated the etiological intracellular agent of the emerging tick-borne infection human granulocytic ehrlichiosis, and has recently identified its leukocyte receptor. He has also been an active clinician and teacher and has directed or participated in major multicenter clinical studies. He has been active in community public health activities, including an environmental health partnership in St. Paul, Minnesota. Among several honors, he has been elected to the American Society for Clinical Investigation.

RENU GUPTA, M.D., holds two positions at Novartis Pharmaceuticals: Head of U.S. Research and Development and Head of Global Cardiovascular, Metabolic and Endocrine G.I. Disorders. As an infectious disease specialist, Dr. Gupta is active in a number of professional societies, including the Infectious Diseases Society of America and the American Society for Microbiology, where she is a member of the committee on education. She is a frequent presenter at the Interscience Conference on Antimicrobial Agents and Chemotherapy and other major infectious disease congresses, and has been published in leading infectious disease periodicals such as the *Journal of Virology*, the *Journal of Infectious Diseases*, and *Antimicrobial Agents and Chemotherapy*. Dr. Gupta received her M.B., Ch.B. from the University of Zambia. Subsequently, she served as Chief Resident in Pediatrics at the Albert Einstein Medical Center and as a Fellow in Infectious Diseases at the Children's Hospital of Philadelphia. She was also a Postdoctoral Fellow in Microbiology at the University of Pennsylvania and the Wistar Institute of Anatomy and Biology, where she conducted research on the pathogenesis of infectious diseases. From 1989 to mid-1998, Dr. Gupta was with Bristol-Myers Squibb Company, where she directed clinical research as well as strategic planning for the Infectious Diseases and Immunology Division. For the past several years, her work has focused on a better understanding of the problem of emerging infections. Dr. Gupta currently chairs the steering committee for the SENTRY Antimicrobial Surveillance Program.

MARGARET A. HAMBURG, M.D., is the immediate past Assistant Secretary for Planning and Evaluation of the U.S. Department of Health and Human Services. Previously, she was the Health Commissioner for the City of New York. She holds appointments as Adjunct Assistant Professor of Medicine at the Cornell University Medical Center and Assistant Professor of Public Health at the Columbia University School of Public Health. In her previous position as special assistant to National Institute of Allergy and Infectious Diseases Director Anthony Fauci, M.D., she played a major role in research administration and policy development in the area of infectious diseases. She serves on the Board of Scientific Counselors of the National Center for Infectious Diseases at the Centers for Disease Control and Prevention. She received her M.D. from Harvard Medical School and completed her internship and residency in internal medicine at New York Hospital/Cornell Medical Center and is board certified in internal medicine. Dr. Hamburg is the author of many scientific articles and is the recipient of numerous awards for distinguished public service.

CAROLE A. HEILMAN, Ph.D., is Director of the Division of Microbiology and Infectious Diseases (DMID) of the National Institute of Allergy and Infectious Diseases (NIAID). Dr. Heilman received her bachelor's degree in biology from Boston University in 1972 and earned her master's degree and doctorate in microbiology from Rutgers University in 1976 and 1979. Dr. Heilman began her career at the National Institutes of Health as a postdoctoral research associate with the National Cancer Institute, where she carried out research on the regulation of gene expression during cancer development. In 1986, she came to NIAID as the Influenza and Viral Respiratory Diseases Program Officer in DMID, and in 1988 she was appointed Chief of the Respiratory Diseases branch, where she coordinated the development of acellular pertussis vaccines. She joined the Division of AIDS as Deputy Director in 1997 and was responsible for developing the Innovation Grant Program for Approaches in human immunodeficiency virus vaccine research. She is the recipient of several notable awards for outstanding achievement. Throughout her extramural career, Dr. Heilman has contributed articles on vaccine design and development to many scientific journals and has served as a consultant to the World Bank and the World Health Organization in this area. She is also a member of several professional societies, including the Infectious Diseases Society of America, the American Society for Microbiology, and the American Society of Virology.

JAMES M. HUGHES, M.D., is Assistant Surgeon General and Director of the National Center for Infectious Diseases (NCID) at the Centers for Disease Control and Prevention (CDC). He was named Deputy Director of NCID in 1988 and became Director of the Center in 1992. He joined CDC as an Epidemic Intelligence Service Officer in 1973, during which time he focused on the epidemiology of food-borne, water-borne, and other diarrheal diseases. Dr. Hughes received his M.D. in 1971 from Stanford University. He is board certified in internal medicine, infectious diseases, and preventive medicine. He is a fellow of the American College of Physicians and the Infectious Diseases Society of America.

SAMUEL L. KATZ, M.D., is the Wilburt C. Davison Professor and chairman emeritus of pediatrics at Duke University Medical Center, and is the immediate past Chairman of the Board of the Burroughs Wellcome Fund. He has concentrated his research on infectious diseases, focusing primarily on vaccine research and development. He is a past chair and a member of the Public Policy Council of the Infectious Diseases Society of America. Dr. Katz has served on a number of scientific advisory committees and is the recipient of many prestigious awards and honorary fellowships in international organizations. Dr. Katz received his M.D. from Harvard Medical School. After his medical internship at Beth Israel Hospital, he completed his pediatrics residency training at the Massachusetts General Hospital and the Boston Children's Hospital. He then became a staff member at Boston Children's Hospital, working with Nobel Laureate John F. Enders, during which time they developed the attenuated measles virus vaccine now used throughout the world. He has chaired the Committee on Infectious Diseases of the American Academy of Pediatrics (the Redbook Committee), the Advisory Committee on Immunization Practices of the Centers for Disease Control and Prevention, the Vaccine Priorities Study of the Institute of Medicine (IOM), and several World Health Organization (WHO) and Children's Vaccine Initiative panels on vaccines and human immunodeficiency virus infections. He is a member of many scientific advisory committees and boards including those of the National Institutes of Health, IOM, and WHO. Dr. Katz's published studies include more than 100 original scientific articles, 60 chapters in textbooks, and many abstracts, editorials, and reviews. He is the coeditor of a textbook on pediatric infectious diseases and has given more than 70 named lectures in the United States and abroad.

MARCELLE LAYTON, M.D., is the Assistant Commissioner for the Bureau of Communicable Diseases at the New York City Department of Health. This bureau is responsible for the surveillance and control of 51 infectious diseases and conditions reportable under the New York City Health Code. Current areas of concern include antibiotic resistance; food-borne, water-borne, and tick-borne diseases; hepatitis C; and biological disaster planning for the potential threats of bioterrorism and pandemic influenza. Dr. Layton received her medical degree from Duke University. She completed an internal medicine residency at the University Health Science Center in Syracuse, New York, and an infectious disease fellowship at Yale University. In addition, Dr. Layton spent 2 years with the Centers for Disease Control and Prevention as a fellow in the Epidemic Intelligence Service, where she was assigned to the New York City Department of Health. In the past, she has volunteered or worked with the Indian Health Service, the Alaskan Native Health Service, and clinics in northwestern Thailand and central Nepal.

CARLOS LOPEZ, Ph.D., is Research Fellow, Research Acquisitions, Eli Lilly Research Laboratories. He received his Ph.D. from the University of Minnesota in 1970. Dr. Lopez was awarded the NTRDA postdoctoral fellowship. After his fellowship he was appointed assistant professor of pathology at the University of Minnesota, where he did his research on cytomegalovirus infections in renal transplant recipients and the consequences of those infections. He was also appointed assistant member and head of the Laboratory of Herpesvirus Infections at the Sloan Kettering Institute for Cancer Research, where his research focused on herpesvirus infections and the mechanisms involved. Dr. Lopez's laboratory contributed to the immunological analysis of the earliest AIDS patients at the beginning of the AIDS epidemic in New York. He is coauthor of one of the seminal publications on this disease as well as many scientific papers and is co-editor of six books. Dr. Lopez has held consultancies with numerous agencies and organizations including the National Institutes of Health, the U.S. Department of Veterans Affairs, and the American Cancer Society.

STEPHEN S. MORSE, Ph.D., is a Professor of Epidemiology at the Columbia University School of Public Health. He was previously a program manager in the Defense Sciences Office at the Defense Advanced Research Projects Agency (DARPA). Dr. Morse was formerly Assistant Professor of Virology at The Rockefeller University. Dr. Morse is a virologist and immunologist with research interests in viral effects on T-lymphocyte development and function, viral zoonoses, and methods for studying viral evolution. He was principal organizer and Chair of the 1989 Conference on Emerging Viruses at the National Institutes of Health and was a member of the Institute of Medicine Committee on Emerging Infections (1990–1992), a member of the Institute of Medicine Committee on Xenograft Transplantation, and Chair of the Microbiology Section of the

New York Academy of Sciences. He was Chair of ProMed (Program for Monitoring Emerging Infections), formed in January 1993 to encourage development of initiatives for anticipating and responding to worldwide emerging infections.

MICHAEL T. OSTERHOLM, Ph.D., M.P.H., is the Chairman and Chief Executive Officer of the Infection Control Advisory Network of Minnesota. Previously, Dr. Osterholm was the State Epidemiologist and Chief of the Acute Disease Epidemiology Section for the Minnesota Department of Health. He is also an adjunct professor of the Division of Epidemiology, School of Public Health, at the University of Minnesota. He has received numerous research awards from the National Institute of Allergy and Infectious Diseases and the Centers for Disease Control and Prevention (CDC). He serves as principal investigator for the CDC-sponsored Emerging Infections Program in Minnesota. He has published more than 140 articles on various emerging infectious disease problems. He is past president of the Council of State and Territorial Epidemiologists and chairs its Committee on Public Health, is a member of the Board of Scientific Counselors, National Center for Infectious Diseases, CDC, and is a member of the National Advisory Committee on Microbial Criteria for Foods, U.S. Department of Agriculture. He recently served as a member of the Committee on the Department of Defense Persian Gulf War Syndrome Comprehensive Clinical Evaluation Program of the Institute of Medicine.

MARC RUBIN, M.D., joined Glaxo Inc. in 1990 as Director of Anti-Infectives. From 1991 to1995 he was Director of Infectious Diseases and Clinical Research, and from 1995 to 1997 was International Director and Vice President of Infectious Diseases and Rheumatology. In 1997, he became Vice President of U.S. Clinical Research and in 1998 became Vice President, Infectious Diseases and Hepatitis, Therapeutic Development and Product Strategy, Glaxo Medical, Regulatory and Product Strategy. He received his B.A. in biology from Cornell University and his medical degree from Cornell University Medical School. Dr. Rubin completed his internship and residency at The Johns Hopkins Hospital, Department of Internal Medicine, and his fellowship and postdoctoral work at the National Cancer Institute. He is board certified in internal medicine, oncology, and infectious diseases.

DAVID M. SHLAES, M.D., Ph.D., is Vice President for Infectious Diseases Research at Wyeth-Ayerst Research. Before joining Wyeth-Ayerst, Dr. Shlaes was professor of medicine at the Case Western Reserve University School of Medicine and Chief of the Infectious Diseases Section and the Clinical Microbiology Unit at the Veterans Affairs Medical Center in Cleveland, Ohio. He has served as a grant reviewer for the U.S. Department of Veterans Affairs Infectious Diseases Merit Review Board and the National Institutes of Health Special Study Section on the Biology of Mycobacteria. He has published widely in peer-reviewed journals, and his interest is in antimicrobial agents and chemotherapy and antibiotic resistance.

JANET SHOEMAKER, is Director of the American Society for Microbiology's Public Affairs Office, a position she has held since 1989. She is responsible for managing the legislative and regulatory affairs of this 42,000-member organization, the largest single biological science society in the world. She has served as principal investigator for a project funded by the National Science Foundation (NSF) to collect and disseminate data on the job market for recent doctorates in microbiology and has played a key role in American Society for Microbiology (ASM) projects, including the production of the ASM *Employment Outlook in the Microbiological Sciences* and *The Impact of Managed Care and Health System Change on Clinical Microbiology.* Previously, she held positions as Assistant Director of Public Affairs for ASM, as ASM coordinator of the U.S./USSR Exchange Program in Microbiology, a program sponsored and coordinated by the National Science Foundation and the U.S. Department of State, and as a freelance editor and writer. She received her baccalaureate, cum laude, from the University of Massachusetts and is a graduate of the George Washington University programs in public policy and in editing and publications. She has served as commissioner to the Commission on Professionals in Science and Technology and as the ASM representative to the ad hoc Group for Medical Research Funding, and she is a member of Women in Government Relations, the Association of Society Executives, and the American Association for the Advancement of Science. She has coauthored published articles on research funding, biotechnology, biological weapons control, and public policy issues related to microbiology.

JOHN D. SIEGFRIED, M.D., is Associate Vice President for Medical, Regulatory and Scientific Affairs at Pharmaceutical Research and Manufacturers of America. Dr. Siegfried is a pediatrician with 25 years in clinical practice and for the past decade has been involved with pharmaceutical research and development in the medical and regulatory affairs section of the R. W. Johnson Pharmaceutical Research Institute. He began his career with the U.S. Public Health Service as a medical officer on the Rosebud and the Redlake Indian Reservations and completed his active pediatric practice as Chief of Pediatrics and Chief of the Medical Staff at the Al Hada Hospital and Rehabilitation Center in Taif, Saudi Arabia. As a volunteer physician, Dr. Siegfried regularly staffs the Whitman-Walker AIDS Clinic in the District of Columbia as well as its clinic for sexually transmitted diseases.

P. FREDERICK SPARLING, M.D., is the J. Herbert Bate Professor of Medicine, Microbiology and Immunology at the University of North Carolina (UNC) at Chapel Hill and is Director of the North Carolina Sexually Transmitted Infections Research Center. Previously he served as Chair of the Department of Medicine and Chair of the Department of Microbiology and Immunology at UNC. He was President of the Infectious Disease Society of American in 1996–1997. He was also a member of the Institute of Medicine's Committee on Microbial Threats to Health (1991–1992). Dr. Sparling's laboratory research is in the molecular biology of bacterial outer membrane proteins involved in pathogenesis, with a major emphasis on gonococci and meningococci. His current studies focus on the biochemistry and genetics of iron-scavenging mechanisms used by gonococci and meningococci and the structure and function of the gonococcal prion proteins. He is pursuing the goal of a vaccine for gonorrhea.

C. DOUGLAS WEBB, JR., Ph.D., received his bachelor's degree in biology from Emory University and his master's degree and doctorate in microbiology from the University of Georgia. He served in the Public Health Service at the Centers for Disease Control and Prevention (CDC) as both a research microbiologist and supervisory microbiologist. After his work at CDC, Dr. Webb went to Pfizer Pharmaceuticals and was involved in the development of ampicillin-sulbactam, carbenicillin, cefoperazone, fluconazole, azithromycin, and trovafloxacin. Dr. Webb is Senior Medical Director in Infectious Diseases Global Marketing at Bristol-Myers Squibb, working on the strategy and development for the anti-infective portfolio including human immunodeficiency virus products.

CATHERINE E. WOTEKI, Ph.D, is immediate former Undersecretary for Food Safety for the U.S. Department of Agriculture. Before receiving Senate confirmation to her present position on July 31, 1997, she served as Acting Undersecretary for Research, Education, and Economics. From 1994 to 1995, she was Deputy to the Associate Director of Science of the Office of Science and Technology Policy. From 1990 to 1994, she was Director of the Food and Nutrition Board, Institute of Medicine, National Academy of Sciences. A biology and chemistry major at Mary Washington College in Fredericksburg, Virginia, she pursued graduate studies in human nutrition at Virginia Polytechnic Institute and State University, Blacksburg, Virginia, and received a Ph.D. in human nutrition. She is a registered dietitian. For 2 years, she performed clinical research in the Department of Medicine of the University of Texas Medical School at San Antonio. She was appointed assistant professor in the Department of Nutrition and Food Science at Drexel University in Philadelphia in 1975. In July 1977, she joined the congressional Office of Technology Assessment as Nutrition Project Director. From 1980 to 1983, she worked for the U.S. Department of Agriculture in two capacities: as leader of the Food and Diet Appraisal Research Group in the Consumer Nutrition Center and as Acting Associate Administrator of the Human Nutrition Information Service. Dr. Woteki was Deputy Director of the Division of Health Examination Statistics, National Center for Health Statistics, U.S. Department of Health and Human Services, from 1983 to 1990. Dr.

Woteki has published 48 articles and numerous technical reports and books on food and nutrition policy and nutrition monitoring. She is the coeditor of *Eat for Life: The Food and Nutrition Board's Guide to Reducing Your Risk of Chronic Disease*. Dr. Woteki is a member of the Institute of Medicine of the National Academies.

STUDY STAFF

JONATHAN R. DAVIS, Ph.D., M.S., is a senior program officer at the Institute of Medicine (IOM). His primary charge is as the Study Director of IOM's Forum on Emerging Infections. Dr. Davis was formerly the Science Officer for the Emerging Infectious Diseases and Human Immunodeficiency Virus/AIDS Program in the U.S. Department of State's Bureau of Oceans and International Environmental and Scientific Affairs. Before his work at the State Department, Dr. Davis was an assistant professor of medicine and head of the Malaria Laboratory at the University of Maryland School of Medicine, where he was the principal and co-principal investigator on grants investigating the fundamental biology of malaria transmission and on the development and testing of candidate malaria vaccines in human volunteers. Dr. Davis has a M.S. in medical entomology from Clemson University and a Ph.D. in immunology and infectious diseases from The Johns Hopkins University School of Hygiene and Public Health. Dr. Davis is an ad hoc reviewer for several professional scientific journals and currently holds adjunct faculty appointments at The Johns Hopkins University School of Hygiene and Public Health, the University of Maryland School of Medicine, and the Uniformed Services University School of the Health Sciences.

VIVIAN P. NOLAN, M.A., is the Research Associate for the Forum on Emerging Infections and for the Roundtable on Research and Development of Drugs, Biologics, and Medical Devices. Before joining the Institute of Medicine (IOM), Ms. Nolan was a Science Assistant in the Division of Environmental Biology at the National Science Foundation (NSF), where she worked on grants administration, research projects, and policy analyses on environmental and conservation biology issues. Ms. Nolan is a recipient of a NSF Directors Award for the policy-oriented, interdisciplinary Water and Watersheds collaborative NSF-U.S. Environmental Protection Agency grants program. Ms. Nolan is pursuing her doctorate degree in environmental science and public policy from George Mason University. Her graduate work has included research and policy analysis on issues including environmental, biodiversity conservation, sustainable development, human health, and emerging and reemerging infectious diseases. In August 1998, she participated in an educational program in Kenya that studied the relationship between ecological degradation and emerging infectious diseases. Ms. Nolan was awarded an M.A. in science, technology, and public policy in 1994 from the George Washington University, and in 1987 she simultaneously earned two bachelor's degrees in international studies and Latin American studies.